IT'S HAPPENING TO ME

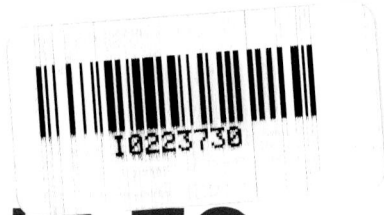

By Rosealine Allen

"One million people commit suicide every year"
World Health Organisation

Published by:
Chipmukapublishing
PO Box 6872
Brentwood
Essex
CM13 1ZT
United Kingdom

www.chipmunkapublishing.com

ISBN 9781847471000

Foreword

Close nit families are interesting, everyone knows. But do they care? This is the life of a person coping with the situation she finds her self in.

This gives real insight into sexual habits in some areas, this book might shock. But it does go one!!

Andrew Latchford
Co founder of Chipmunkapublishing Ltd

CONTENTS

Chapters

Chapter 1: One Love

My earliest memory is of my mum and dad fighting. We lived in a flat on a council estate in Hackney. I remember them shouting at each other and then coming to blows, my mum trying to gouge my dad's eyes out. I was crying and my sister Claudia picked me up and took me out of the bedroom where I was. I must have been about three years old. It was 1970. Can't remember what happened after that.

Life at 8 Samuel House was eventful. Everybody on the Haggerston estate new each other. Beyond my relations, it was like living in one big happy family. We were a multitude of cultures, languages and colour. There were the Martins (of St. Lucian origin like us), the Henrys (they were coolies, I'm not sure which island they were from), the Goggins (white British), Valerie and Barbara (white British), the Hursts (our next door neighbours, white British), the Picketts (Guyanese), Jungle Juice (whose real name was Alex), Rosanna (Italian), Dasos (Greek) and Mad Mary (Irish) of those I can remember. I had seven other siblings, four of us were born here and five born in St Lucia, the first Pauline having died at the age of 8 or 9yrs of cancer. The St. Lucian half of the family were from oldest to youngest – Annabel, Curtis, Francesca and Justine. Just outside the estate was a canal (the Grand Union Canal) and over the bridge of this canal was Laburnum Court where Annabel lived with my nieces Dorothy, Tamara, Jessica and Yvette. The last and final addition to her family was Kevin, her son.

I shared a room with Claudia, Preston and Payton, the younger and English half of the family. My sister and I had bunk beds; my brothers shared a double bed. There was a spare room at the end of the hall, next to my mum and dad's room. We all thought it was haunted. When people visited, they slept in that room. I remember Curtis spooked after sleeping in there one night talking about an elderly white lady appearing by the side of his bed. As he reached out to touch her, she disappeared. On another occasion my sister Francesca while visiting us slept in there. She woke up in the middle of the night to find that she couldn't move or scream. She was pinned down. That was enough to keep the rest of us away from that room for good. It added impact to an event which happened in our room one night. Most nights, once we were all in bed, Claudia would tell us ghost stories. On this particular occasion, it was my turn to switch the light off. As I was small, I had to jump up to reach the switch. I did that and then jumped into my bottom bunk. Claudia began the story, talking slowly to create an eerie atmosphere. I would hang onto her every word, my heart beating ferociously in anticipation. You see she often, after a few sentences, would let out a scream, just to see and hear us jump fearful yet excited by the suspense. Anyway, she did that and we were just getting over the adrenaline rush when the light came on. All by itself. We couldn't run out of that room fast enough, straight into the living room where my mum and dad were watching TV.

I was nicknamed 'Dolly'. My face was the centre of Curtis (when he visited) and Preston's affections. Daily I was plastered with wet sloppy kisses from them on my cheeks while they asked me how I was or what I was doing.

When I protested Preston with a smirk on his face would tell me to shut up, and call me a stupid bit of plastic. Inevitably I'd go complaining to my mum crying who would scream at my brother in a piercing shrill to leave me alone. One day Preston was babysitting Tesaces' (a relative from my mothers side) son Keith and myself. He had a box of matches, and one by one he lit them blew them out and put them to Keith's cheeks. He also heated the shovel handle in the open fire we had in the living room and put it on my arm. He was about 10yrs old then. When my mum got back she gave him the beating of his life. I think that's when she busted his eye with a belt buckle. It was some time after this that he decided to move out, and in with my sister Francesca who lived in Bow.

We were brought up as Catholics. On Saturday mornings my brother Payton and I were sent to catechism. I hardly remember anything about it except singing hymns and seeing the nuns dressed in their nun's habits. We found it so boring that sometimes we would go to Saturday morning cinema for children instead. I made my First Holy Communion with my nieces Tamara and Dorothy. I loved it. Claudia did my hair in ringlets and we had white dresses, veils and shoes just like at a wedding ceremony. It was one of the few occasions on which I had to go to church. The best thing about it was the party and food in the church hall afterward. I didn't really understand the ceremony. While we were preparing for it at Saturday School the nuns said we might be asked questions by the priest. This made me nervous, as I thought I'd get them wrong and they wouldn't allow me to go through with the ceremony, which would have really disappointed my mum. However the priest seemed just as eager to get us through it as my mum because when he asked a question, he answered it himself.

Tamara, Dorothy, Jessica and I spent a lot of time together. It was brilliant. When we weren't playing out we were pretending to be Charlie's Angels with cardigans on our heads (in mock mimicry of their hair) and feigned American accents. We argued over which of the Angels we were going to be and had discussions about which of them were best. One day Dorothy, Vernon Pickett, Gabriela (my sister Justine's daughter) and myself went into mad Mary's flat after she'd moved out. She lived in the block adjacent to Samuel House. We found a mattress, some blankets and pillows, and decided to make a camp. Now the door handle to the room we were in was broken, but I had worked out how we could shut it and open it again. We arranged the mattress, blankets and pillows and I shut the door. When I tried to open it again, it wouldn't open. Panic struck as we each took our turn trying frantically to open it. This room was facing the Grand Union Canal in a flat on the first floor. Separating the canal from the flat was a minor road (not frequently used) and a communal lawn. We opened the window, took a look at the drop down and started crying. We wondered how we were going to get out because if our parents caught us in there, we would get beats. We decided we'd have to jump, but every time we looked out of the window we recoiled burbling we couldn't do it. We threw everything we had on the lawn beneath the window, which we hoped would cushion our landing. Dorothy went first ending up with whiplash. I dropped Gabriela out next, then only about three years old, who was crying hysterically. Dorothy caught her. Then me. Vernon, despite our telling him that he would be alright, just looked down at us tears streaming down his face. 'Come on!' we shouted, 'we haven't got all day.' Justine, came along at one point on her way to my sister Annabel's place, and asked us what we were doing. Luckily she was too far away from us to see exactly what we were doing. We ran over to her so that she couldn't see Vernon, put her mind at rest and when she was out of sight, went back to Vernon. Well, Vernon didn't have to jump after all. A white man came by and helped him down. We couldn't believe his luck. We walked home flushed with our cricked necks and unable to contain ourselves at what we had just been through.

Young as we were, sexual encounters were commonplace. Claudia was dating someone called David, and at night in the porch, they would make out. My mother would go berserk. She would yell at Claudia telling her to come upstairs saying she was nasty and she even went as far as throwing a bucket of urine downstairs at them. At nursery, Dorothy, myself, and our friends Claire (an Irish girl whose mother worked at our school), Lawrence (white British) and Vernon, were always playing kiss chase. Claire was my best friend at school and although we weren't allowed to eat sweets in school her mother who worked at the school, often snuck us some. She went to live in the USA before I left Laburnum and that was the end of that friendship. It didn't even cross my mind that we could have kept in touch as pen pals. There was a girl at school when I was about 8yrs old called Manuella. She was Greek or Turkish I can't remember which, but she got pregnant at 8 or 9yrs old by her uncle. She stopped coming to school after that.

When Dorothy (the same age as me) came round to my place, we would pretend to be lovers. We would make out in my bedroom when no one else was around. Of course, I imagine they all thought we were playing with my toys. We were caught in the act by Francesca once. She dragged me by the arm into the living room where everyone was watching TV and told them all what we were doing. I was crying hysterically, probably terrified I'd get beaten, and Dorothy managed to escape the whole scene. I think my sister sent her home. We didn't do that again after that. There were sexual incidents with my brother Payton and his friends too. There had been a fire in one of the flats in our block and Payton, his friend Dasos and me went in there exploring. My brother tried to put his penis into my vagina and had his friend observe the whole thing. He was two years older than me. When we left, Preston saw us and asked us where we'd been. There were patches of soot on our clothes. Without us answering him he said smirking to himself obviously enlightened, "I know where you've been. Don't go there again otherwise I'll tell mummy." It was as if he knew what we had been doing. On another occasion Errol and Tony Henry, my brother and I were listening to music in their front room. Somehow, I started dancing for them. They leered at me and lifted my skirt, but I was completely absorbed in the dancing. Also, Tony came up to see Payton one day, but he wasn't in. I was in my nightdress as it was late. For some reason we were hitting each other, and Tony got closer and closer to me with each tap until he was rubbing his groin against me, against the wall. He was a year or two older than me.

Our summer holidays on the Haggerston Estate were filled with activities arranged by a group of hippies. They organized fun runs that entailed following instructions at set points and carrying out a request over a distance of some miles in the local area. The first to arrive home got a prize. There were singing competitions and art classes. One summer, they planned a camping trip. I begged my mum to let me go. One of the girls that was going even went to my mum and told her she would look after me. My mum resounded a finite *NO*, and that was that. Claudia and Preston said it was fantastic when they got back. There were ghosts, they went swimming in a lake, and were chased by a bull.

Football was extremely popular on our estate too. Matches were arranged with the Hillcot mob. These were mainly Jamaicans who lived in the neighbouring estate called Hillcot. The games were not restricted to men. Claudia use to play with them. We also played bulldog on the grassy area on the estate and painted murals on the walls. Valerie, who lived in mad Mary's block, invited me into her place once. She made sugar and tomato ketchup sandwiches with the butter spread so thick it looked like cheese. They were *disgusting*! Barbara one of our neighbours, had epilepsy and sometimes she would be out playing, and have an epileptic fit. I just stared in amazement. There was a deaf and dumb girl too. She was black. I don't remember much about her, just that trying to communicate with her was difficult. Bunny (a nickname I believe), Leroy and Vernon's dad, had a party one day. It was for adults only. I was sent on an errand by my mum to that party, and while there, Bunny gave me some of his drink. I don't know what it was, but as soon as I left to go home, my head started spinning. I jumped down the stairs and fell down at the bottom of them. I don't know how I got home, but I did.

Sometimes we would climb through a gap in the railings fencing the canal from the road and sit at the side of the canal playing with the water snails. We weren't allowed by the canal, as there were rumours that if you fell in, the weeds would drag you under and you would drown. Donna Martin was my best friend on the estate. Every summer for a few days, flying ants would swarm the estate. They were awful, as they got in our hair, eyes and on our clothes. I remember Donna and I got an old pram and a stick one day and took it in turns pushing each other across the tarmac in front of the flats and used the stick to kill every flying ant we saw.

Every evening in the summer an ice-cream van came round. He would give me an ice cream for however much money I had. His was the best ice cream I have ever tasted! It was cream coloured and tasted as though it had real cream in it. Not like ice cream today. My nieces and I used to steal from the sweetshop too. One of us would keep the shopkeeper occupied, and the rest of us would stuff our pockets with penny sweets and chewing gums. Suffice it to say, In spite of the fact that we were poor, I got some fashionable clothes and shoes. Mini skirts, a flared backless cat suit and a pair of clogs. Francesca made her own clothes and sometimes she'd make some for me. Also, Claire's mother use to give me Claire's cast-offs and once a week, like a ritual from the Middle Ages and looking as though he'd come out of a coal mine, the rag 'n' bone man would come calling for 'any old iron!' We gave him our old clothes, pots and pans. In addition, 'Jungle

Juice' was a black man, dark in complexion who always wore black clothes. We would tease him, calling up to him in his flat. When he opened the door we would scream and run away. He was a great artist though. He painted a really beautiful picture one summer.

Sunday mornings my brothers played money up the wall. My Sunday best, a pink and white polka dot dress had holes under the arms and in one of the tiers. Both my mum and dad were working as unskilled labourers. My dad in a furniture factory, and my mum as a catering assistant in a hospital. Sometimes, I went to meet my dad especially on a Friday, at the end of the working day. He would grumble about his employer, walking extremely quickly and barely noticing my presence. I don't remember when he stopped work, but he gambled on the horses a lot. He would get up extremely early, buy a paper and a packet of sweets for me and then spend the next hour or two studying the races. Occasionally he'd get me to choose a horse for him thinking I would bring him good luck. Mum, through all of this, did *everything*. The double bed in our room had a metal frame with metal springs which was very old. It was crawling with what my mum called 'pinnes' (bed bugs). She said they suck your blood. Every so often she would take the mattress off the bed and pour boiling hot water over the springs and frame.

We had our fair share of pets too. A black dog called Bruce who would wake us up for school in the morning by jumping on the beds and licking our faces. We had a couple of budgerigars. A blue one called Bill and a green one called Jim. They were kept on a huge old wooden table my mum kept in the hall. Once a week, I would let them out into my mums 'best' room. We kept goldfish on this table too. I use to have nightmares that featured that wooden table. I would be standing at one end of it and there would be a witch on the other side. Ever so slowly, she would draw closer and closer to me. I was terrified and tried to run but my feet were stuck to the ground and I would just stare at her getting closer the terror welling up inside me. When she was just about to touch me I would lash out, arms flailing and then start running for my life. I ran straight to Annabel's place and when she opened the door to me she had the witches eyes too, so I kept running. Every family member I came into contact with turned on me with the witches eyes, and then I'd wake up.

Annabel had a dog called Elsa. She was really wild because my nieces and nephew tormented her. She would chew all the gussets on their knickers from the laundry basket and airing cupboard as if she were getting her own back on them, but she got serious beatings for it. Whenever my brother and I were at Annabel's place we always wanted what she was cooking. Its not that we weren't fed, everything just seemed more appetizing at her place. So Payton and I would sit patiently hoping she would dish some out to us. Mmmm, apple pie and custard! Sometimes she did, but most times she sent us home telling us to go home for our dinner. On the way home, we would moan about how mean she was, saying that her kids were always eating at our place. I remember one thing she did give us and that was senna tea. She told us it was good for us and it would clear our skin. It was the most foul tasting tea I had ever tasted. So there we all sat sipping senna tea and a couple of minutes later, we were fighting each other for the toilet. For a while, I don't remember what the circumstances were, but my uncles daughter Pinky, was staying with Annabel. She wasn't really welcome. It was just a makeshift arrangement. Dorothy told me Pinky came on her period once and bled all over the bathroom floor, when Dorothy went to use the bathroom she slipped in it. It didn't do much for her popularity with Annabel and her kids. My mum loved Dorothy with a passion unrivalled by the love she gave to any of her own children. I think this was partly because Dorothy was plump, and mum was on the larger side too. I would get so angry with my mum as a result of this and often had to remind her that *I* was her daughter, not Dorothy. She'd just laugh at me.

At some point I got a toy cash till from my mum or dad. I use to set up a stall on the estate selling everything that I no longer wanted. In particular I sold pens that my dad got from the bookmakers every time he went. I sold them for a penny each. Surprisingly, people actually bought things from me, and I'd spend the money on a feast of sweets usually. Justine lived not a great distance away. She lived on the Holly Street Estate which was back then adjacent to Glebe Road. Gabriela was born in 1972. I spent a lot of time at Justine's as a child. I was there with my mum and Tesace once who had brought a cake containing some sort of seed. A voice told me not to eat it, as she was a witch. Tesace urged me to eat some cake, but I just stared at her suspiciously, telling her I didn't like the seeds. At the back of Justine's flat was an adventure playground. Dorothy and I would spend lots and lots of time there climbing on the frames and swinging on the swings. It was great fun. On my 6th birthday, my sisters Francesca and Justine got my ears pierced for me, and took me to the Wimpy bar for something to eat. It was a real treat. While they gassed on, I gobbled my Wimpy hamburger.

Just before we left the Haggerston Estate our dog Bruce went missing. We searched everywhere for him until we heard from someone that they'd seen a white couple walking away with a black dog. He was such a good clever dog that we were really saddened by losing him. And then we moved. The council moved everyone out of the estate, because they wanted to renovate it. We were housed in the neighbouring borough of Tower Hamlets.

Chapter 2: Differences

It was 1975 when we moved to Firth House in Bethnal Green. I think we moved in the summer. There was a rose bed at the back of the flats with a communal lawn and a concrete area separated from the road by a parapet at the front. We lived on the ground floor. In the winter we discovered that the flat was damp. The walls were blackened by it in the bathroom, my brother Payton's room was covered by it in one corner, and in Claudia's room the clothes cupboard was affected by it. It ruined our clothes. The kitchen sink was surrounded by a wooden draining board beneath which was a cupboard. There were holes in the draining board where the tap pipes went down into the cupboard. Particularly at night woodlice would come through the holes, like they were coming up for air. I hated it! The cupboard in my sister's bedroom was crawling with silverfish too. This also made my skin crawl. Across the road was the remainder of an army barracks. My brother and I would climb over the wall into it and search out spider's webs. We'd find insects to throw on them just so that we could see the spider come and wrap it up in its web.

Claudia was tall, slim and attractive. The St. Lucian half of the family teased her about her height when she was younger and as a result, she stopped talking to them. Anyway, she tried to get into modelling and use to practice her walks in the hall in her many different outfits. She was always dieting, or she would eat, and then throw it up. I figured if she needed to diet as slim as she was, then I needed to diet too, although with me it was often just lip service, at that time. She got a sewing machine from Annabel at one point, and she started to make her own things. She made me a black and white speckled pencil skirt, and a black top that had a belt, to match it. I thought I was the *business*! We use to practice yoga together and both Payton and she were good at drawing. Her boyfriend David use to play the guitar and when I learned to play the recorder, we use to do duets. It didn't work out with modelling. She said they wanted her to cut her hair short which she really didn't want to do. There were other things too, but at that time I think they were too difficult to articulate.

So at the age of 8yrs, I began a new school. It was called Columbia School and I was one of only a few black children there. They use to tease me about my hair, which my mum combed into plaits, and call me 'carrots'. Mark Priest and Stephen Saunders were two of the cleverest in the class as they were from different social backgrounds to the rest but I think that they were impressed at how clever I was. I participated in just about every extra-curricular activity there was. Miss Peddar led netball. I always played in the position of 'goal attack'. Mr Webb took us for rounders in my final year at school. He was also my final year teacher. There was a tournament at Victoria Park on one occasion. Great fun! He also taught gymnastics after school which I wasn't much good at, but I kept it up anyway. Mrs White taught country dancing at lunchtimes, and there was a chess club which I attended occasionally, more for observation than participation because to be honest, I wasn't very good. The head of the school Mr Hawes was in charge of music and taught badminton. I was good at badminton because I played on Sundays with my brothers and sisters and I *loved* our music sessions. As well as playing the recorder, my mum bought me a tenor, similar to a recorder but a bit larger, and Mr Hawes taught me how to play that too. There was a percussion music group and a choir and those that excelled in music had sessions with Mr Hawes listening to classical music, which he was very passionate about.

My first teacher when I joined Columbia, was remarkably sensitive. She reminded me of a Dutch girl. She often wore her hair in two plaits and she wore clogs. We had terrapins in the classroom. Miss Peddar, my teacher between the ages of 9 to 10yrs had ginger hair. She was partially Scottish, although she didn't have a Scottish accent. We grew plants in her class, avocado seeds and beans, and I remember having hand writing lessons. When we had mastered joined up writing we were allowed to write with fountain pens. Mr Webb was a cockney although his accent was a bit softer than that of a typical cockney. He was tall and thin with glasses. Mrs White was from the north although her accent was wearing off, and Mr Hawes was well built with a moustache and mousy brown hair. I didn't have many friends at Columbia school. I remember an occasion when two children from Nigeria joined the school. They were brother and sister, the boy being older than the girl. It was the end of playtime, and we were queuing up in our classes as we usually did, to go back into the classrooms. The Nigerian boy pushed in front of me with his sister. I told him I was there first, and stood in front of him. He pushed me out of the way. I was so incensed and don't ask me where it came from, but I called him a *nigger*. Well, we were both pulled aside and sent up to Mr Hawes' office where we were severely berated. Mr Hawes said to me, "Now that was a stupid thing to call him wasn't it?" I was silent. I suppose calling him that came from my mother who one by one saw my sisters give themselves to black men who didn't care for them, and didn't respect them. She was really bitter about this. There was another incident one lunchtime when I was playing 'dibs' with a few of the girls from my class too. I saw Steven Bristow (a white boy) kicking Lorna Rhoden (a black girl) in the stomach against the wall. I couldn't believe it. I ran over to them and pushed him away and asked him what he thought was doing. He said, "It's nothing to do with you Mitchell". We started arguing until one of the teachers came over to find out what the problem was.

The school put on a show every year. The first one was the Wizard of Oz. Ruth (a Jewish girl who was short and on the plump side) and myself were to take it in turns at being Dorothy. However I felt she was much better at it than me so decided to let her play Dorothy every night of the show. Mr Hawes asked me if she'd bullied me into allowing her to play Dorothy. Anyway, I played Dorothy's friend and had Mark Staples (partly Italian) as my father. In the show I had to kiss him on the cheek. Some of the girls in my class came up to me afterward and said, "You're so lucky. You have to kiss *Mark Staples*." It was then that I realized he was the school don. Also, one of the few friends I had was a girl called Diane, but after a while she decided we had nothing in common and brought the friendship to a close. I ended up becoming pals with Ruth and Laura. During our breaks we played 'dibs' and 'jacks'. We went to the Isle of Wight when I was in Miss Peddar's class too.

I got travel sick, and was throwing up every couple of hours. But I remember being by the sea which was really beautiful and being blown by the fresh sea air. Soon Mark Staples and Simon Grosvenor (his friend), became the apple of my eye. Surprise, surprise! When I found out where they lived, I use to go and hang out there with Dorothy hoping to catch a glimpse of them.

We had two piano accompanists at school. First was a Chinese woman who every few minutes would plaster her hands with Johnson's baby lotion. The second was Miss Mitchell. She was English. I remember asking her how old she was when she had started playing the piano, to which she responded 18yrs. I reckoned if I started playing as soon as I started secondary school I would be as good as her before I reached the age of 18. We had a school fair every year too. Mr Hawes was on a stall where he had his face and hands poking through a stocks and pillory and you had to throw wet sponges at him. I won the raffle competition at that fair. I also entered a cake making competition one Easter. I covered my cake with Smarties saying 'Happy Easter', but I didn't win.

After school my brother and I spent our time around the flats. We got to know everyone very quickly. First were the Sonnies whose parents were of St. Lucian origin like ours. There was Rosemary, Sharon and Lorraine. They had a brother, but he was much older and so didn't hang out with us. Rosemary was also a bit older and was fat, but had a two dimensional shape, that is she was more or less flat. She went out with a white guy called Steve who had a twin brother. He doted on her and they were often seen clinched in unbridled displays of passion. There was

Simone Butler and her brother Nathan. They lived in South Africa for a few years as her father was a member of the army, but they were white. There was Winston Gordon (whose parents were from Jamaica). His mother worked at the same hospital as my mum. Winston was a bit of a joker. He would mimic the stereotype of black people in the way he laughed and spoke. Andrew Wallace was a coolie who was adopted by Oliver Millett's mother. She was a nurse like the Sonnie's mother. He was thin with an athletic build and curly black hair. Shafkot and Arthur were Moslem Pakistanis. Arthur (a girl) had an arranged marriage when she was 13 or 14, and had a baby when she was 15 years old. The Angles were a family of four boys whose parents were from Dominica. At about this time I became preoccupied with boys. It was like an obsession. Lorraine and I used to go '*man hunting*' (a term coined by Lorraine). We would walk the streets looking for good looking men and ogle them.

I don't recall how this came about, but Dorothy (when she came round to our place), Simone, and myself formed a group called the '*Women's Daredevils*'. We would seek out feats that each member had to perform. And each feat became a burden until you performed the activity. We were young, courageous and careless, I suppose. The activities included jumping from high walls onto a concrete surface, or standing on a shed and jumping onto the grass below, or jumping from a garden wall across a clearing onto a shed. No matter how frightening the feat, we all always carried it out. We must have aggravated a lot of people at that time, particularly when we played 'knock down ginger'. I remember once, we were playing 'knock down ginger' on a new neighbouring estate. We were running around laughing hysterically, opening and closing doors when we heard police sirens quite nearby. To get out of the part of the estate we were in, we had to climb up a ladder onto a roof and then jump down on the other side. Simone was the first escapee. Dorothy went to go next, but I was so terrified that I'd get caught alone, that I pulled her back down the ladder. Anyway we managed to get home without being caught but I was a nervous wreck afterward. During the summer holidays Dorothy, Simone and I would go to Spitalfields City Farm, when it was next to Brick Lane. It was *wonderful*! We mucked out the pony 'Jubilee' and the donkey, groomed them and fed them. There were goats, geese and chickens too. We were filmed on a programme about farming by I think it was the BBC at one stage. An artist was commissioned to paint a mural on the farm wall also, which we all participated in. We had water fights back at the estate too during which we swore at each other like troopers while in fits of laughter, and when we weren't doing that we were roller-skating around London. We went all the way to Hyde Park on our skates once. I had a bicycle also, on which I'd circle our block of flats when I had nothing else to do.

Gabriela was always staying at our place. I loved having her over because it gave me the opportunity to play mum. She was like a younger sister. My dad used to bring her over because he used to say he felt sorry for her. Justine was always telling her off. She had many peculiarities about her. Apart from being tiny, she developed a severe squint. I called her 'Blinky' as a result. Whenever we were out, if she saw any dogs muck on the ground, she would cross to the other side of the street rather than pass it, and she was a remarkably fastidious eater. I liked giving her a wash and dressing her up. My mum use to call her 'Chichick femme' (meaning 'little woman'). We were getting ready to go swimming once so she had a swimming costume on and was playing with one of my dolls. She went to the toilet and then came out again without the doll. I asked her where the doll was. I can't remember what she answered, but I discovered that she had broken it and hidden it in the crutch of her swimming costume. To say the least, I was *outraged*. I stripped her naked and pulled her into the porch of our flats so as to make a public display of her. Awful! She was crying hysterically. Poor Gabriela. We use to go to a play centre in the summer sometimes. I remember winning a modelling competition they held there. I don't know how, because on the day that I had won, my hair hadn't even been combed. I entered Jessica in a fancy dress competition at the same play centre. Jessica had a different dad to Tamara and Dorothy. He was a coolie, so she had really soft hair. I dressed her up as a Hawaiian girl. Her grass skirt consisted of black and white chequered cloth (that was all I had), she wore one of my bikini tops, had a flower in her hair and I put make up on her. She didn't win, but she did get a runners up prize.

My brother Payton had a bit of a wild streak. Not only did he get into lots of fights, but he was always stirring things up between people. When 'trick or treaters' or carol singers knocked at our door, he always did something ridiculous. On one occasion I answered the door to some 'trick or treaters' on Halloween embarrassed that we didn't have anything to give them. My brother, seeing who it was, then went back into the living room, feigned a St. Lucian accent and shouted, "bring me some hot water to

throw over whoever is at the door!" I felt the laughter
mixed with embarrassment welling up inside of me, so I
shut the door and then burst into fits of giggles. We
decided we were going to make a movie once, a black
version of the West Side Story. I was to write the script. I
do recall starting it, but I'm not sure what happened after
the first few pages. Perhaps it was just a little too
ambitious for us at that time. Often Payton and myself
would go to see Chrissy and Maria, Curtis's children from
his marriage with a woman called Teresa. At least that's
what she claims, but he denies. We got up to all sorts of
mischief. They lived on an estate next to Francesca's flats
in Bow. There was a pub called the 'Bombay Crab' where
they had nude dancing. We would peak through the door,
shout something rude at the punters and then scarper. We
also went blackberry picking along the River Lea near to
Bow Creek. Payton and I would take the blackberries
home and make black berry pies. They were *delicious*! I
stayed with Francesca one Christmas. She had a couple of
friends in her block, Seneva (an Irish woman) and Ramie
(an Indian man). They were having an affair. Anyway,
Seneva bought me a doll for Christmas. Unlike my
parents, she wrapped all her gifts, and put them under the
Christmas tree. That seemed to make them all the more
exciting for me. Francesca had a son, Terrence about the
same age as Gabriela and a grey Siamese cat called
'Smokey'. Some mornings the cat would kill a bird and
leave it on her doorstep, and when I was sitting in the
living room, it sat on my lap chose a spot on my nightdress
and would lick that one spot, all the while purring and
flexing and unflexing its claws. Francesca was seeing a
guy called Todd at the time. Not Terrence's dad. They

weren't getting on that well. He was a mixed race, Chinese and Jamaican. She had a daughter with him called Sabrina.

Back at home our first cousins lived just down the road from us. They were my dad's brother Anthony's children. Alan, June, Emmanuel and Nelson from oldest to youngest in that order. Nelson and Emmanuel new all the latest dances, so Payton and myself would often go to them to learn from them. We danced to all the latest soul and dance music of that era. I remember seeing June's picture in a new black hairdresser called 'Joseph's' on Bethnal Green Road. She had her hair relaxed. She looked really *good*. Occasionally my mum would take me to Paddington to see my uncles and aunts, her brothers and sisters. There was always plenty of food spread before us. In particular I remember three of my first cousins from this period. Mark, uncle Ravino's son. My aunt Mary was always scolding him. She made me laugh. There was Liza (pronounced Leeza), uncle John's daughter. Uncle John would always give us some money to buy some sweets when I was there. He said she was very naughty. Then there was Joycelyn, my aunt Vero's daughter. I remember she was having problems studying. She said whenever she read something, she couldn't remember it, no matter how many times she went over it. She was really distressed by it. Sometimes I would go and visit Claudia and David who were living in Well Street, Hackney. They had a gorgeous dog called 'Benji' who was a cross between a golden retriever and a husky of sorts, but very difficult to handle. We had a barbecue in their back yard once and I became pals with their Greek neighbours.

It was the late 70's and the National Front had a strong following in Tower Hamlets. I remember they marched down Bethnal Green Road on two occasions. Whenever I heard they were marching, I ran home terrified. In 1978, the movie 'Grease' came out and we couldn't think about anything else. All we girls wanted to be Olivia Newton John, regardless of the fact that she was white. Simone got the whole kit. She had a mass of blonde curls and was extremely slim. She got the skin tight black trousers and a boob tube and what with her hair, she said people were saying she looked like Olivia Newton John's sister. We sang the songs in the streets and in partners played the parts of Olivia Newton John and John Travolta in the love shack.

I fancied Andrew Wallace like mad, but nothing happened. You see everyone was terrified of my brother because of his reputation, Andrew included. So he ignored my attempts at flirting with him. We were in the park on the estate once, Andrew, Jessica and myself and it was a bit cold, not so cold that I couldn't bare it. Anyway I asked Andrew if I could wear his jacket just to see if he had any feelings for me whatsoever, and he laughed and shouted, "No chance!" Jessica burst into fits of laughter. I had a very brief encounter with Desmond Angle, all supervised by my brother. We kissed in a garage once while a couple of my other nieces kissed his brothers. Payton had a girlfriend called Clare. I almost worshipped the ground she walked on, she was so clever and attractive. She had a short afro and was tall and slim. She went to Central Foundation School. When it was my time to go to secondary school, I begged my mum to let me go to Clare's school, but she was adamant that I was going to

Haggerston school for girls because it was closer to us. Anyway, Clare and my brother didn't last long, and the last I heard of her was that she got pregnant at age 15yrs.

One day I was sent on an errand by my mum to Mrs Angles place. She use to cook black puddings, and sell them to the local Caribbean community. So I was on my way to buy some for my mum. As I was walking past Daneford School, a white man stopped by me in his car and asked me for directions to a place locally. I didn't have a clue so said to him, "Sorry, I don't know". He then said, "look love," and looked down at his crutch where he was holding his penis in his hand. I ran for my life, all the way to Mrs Angles place, and told them about my ordeal.

Mum's cooking was *delicious*. In the winter time she cooked oats porridge and 'Timmy' (which is cornmeal porridge) with plenty of spices and sugar. Sunday mornings we had a full English breakfast. At night time she would make ginger tea and hot chocolate with real cocoa. My favourite meal was lamb with mint sauce and boiled potatoes. On Good Friday's we weren't allowed to eat meat and there was a tradition (at least among St. Lucians) of cooking fishcakes, made with saltfish. One day, my mum had the kitchen windows open and as she was cooking with her huge pots characteristic of the West Indian people of her generation, steam was bellowing out of the window. I was playing out front, and a couple of white boys came up to me and seeing the pots through the window said, "Is your mum a witch?" Deeply offended, I retaliated, "No she is not!" All I could think of was the association they were making between a thing I perceived as terrifying, and my mother who was black.

When my mum washed my hair, it was a fight to comb it through afterward. I hated having my hair washed because of this. Combing the tangles out was a nightmare even though she put grease in it, of various kinds, to lubricate it. In the winter when she used coconut oil, it would harden and show up as white specs in my hair. It was *shameful*, but I had long hair for a black girl back then.

Every so often there would be coach trips to the fairground. I remember going to Margate and Blackpool. There would be a sea of black faces on the coach and the air was permeated by the smell of rice, peas and chicken. This didn't do much for my travel sickness. At the faigrounds, we use to seek out the scariest and most dangerous rides; the 'big dipper' and the 'wild mouse' are two that I remember, and we stuffed our faces with candyfloss, and doughnuts. I use to forego my dinner sometimes for a couple of chocolate bars. I was addicted to 'Marathon' bars, as was Lorraine. Sometimes, Andrew's older brother would have a disco for all of us around the flats. He lived on the estate too, and had tons and tons of records. All the latest in soul and dance.

Although we lived on the same estate, I slept at Simone's place once. Her parents were quite strict, and if she did wrong, she got a good hiding for it. Her dad use to beat her mum too and unlike my mum and dad, I don't think her mum fought back. Simone wasn't allowed to eat anything from the kitchen without asking her mother first, and when she had biscuits, she only had two whereas I'd get through a whole packet in an evening. Not surprisingly our physiques were very different. We played 'Scrabble', and her mother use to point to me as a model child, saying to her, "Why can't you be like Rosie?" Simone said she had servants when she lived in South Africa. She had a nasal tone to her voice, and when she breathed, it was like she was struggling to get air through her nostrils her nose was so narrow and pointed, that she used to breathe through her mouth. Well, I thought, as Simone had allowed me to stay at her place, I should reciprocate. What a nightmare that was. I suddenly noticed everything that was wrong with our flat. How unclean it was, how poor the furniture was. I spent the whole evening cleaning up and left Simone to watch TV. I was *so ashamed*! I tried to wipe the damp off of the walls in the bathroom. When she left the next day I told my mum we should decorate.

I had chicken pox twice. It was *awful*! When the spots itched, it was nice scratching them, until they formed scabs. Then, scratching them was painful. I got some 'calamine' lotion from the doctor, but that didn't help much. When Simone got chicken pox she said her mum gave her cold baths to cool her body temperature, smothered the spots in 'calamine' lotion and dressed her in a loose fitting nightdress so as not to irritate the spots. One night, at about 3 a.m. I was woken by a whizzing pain through one of my back teeth. It was a tooth I had a filling in only a few weeks earlier. I screamed out in pain, and then it stopped only to come back a couple of hours later. Like a woman in labour about to give birth, the distance between each episode of pain got shorter and shorter. At about 8.30 a.m. I made my way to the dentist with my mum a reluctant escort. The pain was unbearable and as soon as the receptionist saw me she showed me through to the dentist who drilled the tooth again, took out the nerve and put another filling in.

In the last few months of being at Columbia School, we sat our 11+ examinations. We were examined in the three R's: reading, writing and arithmetic. I got top grades in all three, 1,1,1. We had a visit from the Head of the first year of Haggerston School. Her name was Mrs Wilby. She was white, but wore dark clothes and had dyed black hair. She was pleasant enough I suppose. And, that was the end of Columbia School, but we continued living at Firth House.

Chapter 3: Puberty

Simone started her period when she was 11 years old. I couldn't *believe* it! Her bust was bigger than mine and although she was much slimmer than me, she was curvaceous. Her breasts were like ripe plums that stuck out slightly to the side and her legs were long and willowy. I on the other hand hardly had a chest, and insensuously what I did have simply pointed straight forward, and my brother said I had footballers legs. I complained to God and asked him why he allowed Simone to have her period before me, not that it got me anywhere. Anyway, that's what I started doing, noticing women's shapes more and comparing myself to them. I'd go to the market with my mum on a Saturday morning and see white girls dressed in figure hugging jeans so that you could see every contour on their bodies. My sister got me a pair of tight jeans eventually and I bought a chiffon shirt to go with them. Most of my clothes though came from a salesman who worked in the Queen Elizabeth Hospital for children with my mum on Hackney Road. Some of his stuff was modern, and some was a bit old fashioned. The rest of my clothes I got from Bethnal Green Market, and the shops along Bethnal Green road. I use to knit too. I made myself a navy blue jersey dress that I thought was really smart when I wore it with blue woolly tights and a belt around the waist.

At school, we wore a grey uniform. My feet were enormous and at that time, it was fashionable for women to have small feet. I struggled to squeeze them into a size 5, but they were begging for a 6 and I was only about 5'3". I thought I looked like '*Sasquatch*'. No matter what I wore I felt as though my feet were protruding as though I had flippers on. I would get huge blisters sometimes because I squeezed my feet into tight fitting shoes. Claudia didn't like the size of her feet either, but at least she had the height to go with big feet! So I started school in September 1978. We were divided into streams, which meant that Ruth and I, having both got top grades in the 11+ exams, were in the same class. We became relatively good friends such that we were always together. There were a few others in our class that we hung out with at breaks and lunchtimes. There was Janice whose parents were Jamaican. She had a mild stammer. There was also Lorraine T. and Cordelia both of who's parents were also from one of the Caribbean islands, Sai Fan Pang who was oriental I think from Hong Kong, and Heather who my brother use to call *guiness* because she had brown / blonde hair. I think she was from Barbados and left to go back there in the second year. She got on with Ruth like a house on fire. They were both so loud and boisterous.

We studied a much wider variety of subjects in the lower half of secondary school than we did at primary school. Mr Sackman took us for music and I found myself developing a crush on him, but I didn't tell anyone. So did Ruth, but she confided in me about hers. Mr Sackman had shoulder length dark hair cut into a bob and wore flared trousers. When I was walking home from school, I use to think he was *watching* me, that he was driving in his car nearby, and watching me walk home. I use to *dread* English lessons because I never knew *what* to say and because Mrs Atkin was extremely *sharp*, in every sense of the word. That is, in the way she walked and spoke. Unlike Mr Sackman, there wasn't a trace of the 60's and 70's about her even though she told us she was a *socialist*. She use to get her son, to mark our English essays, and her husband was an examiner. Painfully, I remember an incident in English where we were discussing marriage and she wanted to know what we thought as a class about the woman taking on her husband's surname. She asked me what *I* thought. I didn't have a clue and said, "You might not like his surname." Can't recall what she said afterward, but I felt so *foolish.* I was so terrified of reading in that class that whenever I was asked to read by Mrs Atkin I would pronounce every single letter in each word. The other girls started calling me a snob as a result. There was an occasion on which I got one of my essays read out to the class by Mrs Atkin too. It was about Christmas in our flat. I cringed all the way through it. But, I must say even though I never excelled in English literature, I *loved* it. I remember Mrs Atkin took us to a poetry conference once, full of girls that were all about our age. They looked and sounded as though they were in finishing school though. One of them had a pet *rat!* Miss Poole took us for French, which was another of my favourite subjects. She was a really *wonderful* teacher who got married in our third year and became Mrs Brookes, and went to live in Barbados with her husband.

There were a couple of week long trips abroad when I was in the lower school. The first was to France. Janice Ruth and I shared a room and we all slept in a double bed. Our hotel was quite near the beech and after our first day there, I got a rash all over my back. Back then I attributed it to the sand, but in retrospect, I think it might have been the heat. There was an incident with some boys on a motorbike. They were chasing us down the stairs to the beach on their bikes. We pretended to be afraid and ran away screaming. Janice on the other hand, stood her ground and gave them an 'if looks could kill' look, and they stopped chasing us after that. In France, we were allowed in pubs back then, so one evening we all went to a pub with Miss Poole and had a glass of 'Orangina'. The French assistant came on the trip with us, and she took us to a creperie where we had crepes with chocolate sauce or jam. The other trip was to various places in Europe. We went through France, Italy, Germany and Austria, of what I can remember. In Austria our hotel was near a lake, so we went swimming there often, it was *so hot*. There were frogs in the water and slime at the lakes edges. It was nice though. One night, Ruth and I got back late as we'd been out on a day trip. It was pitch black so we went to switch on the lamp and realized the bulb had been taken out. We figured it must have been Janet Lacey and Debbie Mitchell who were in the next room. I shouted '*Beasts*!' And then we heard the faint titter of Janet and Debbie next door. To top it all, there was a noisy fly buzzing around the room and near my ears. One of the teachers came in and asked us what the fuss was. We told her what had happened but she simply told us to settle down as it was late, and she opened the window to let the fly out.

My first name was the cause of much contention in secondary school. On my birth certificate it was spelt Roselyn, but when my dad spelt it out for me when I was younger, he use to spell it Rosealine pronounced Roslyn. Ruth, use to call me by my name and pronounce the 'a' in the middle, and instead of saying 'lyn' at the end said 'line', Roz-a-line. Some of the teachers seemed baffled too and were always questioning me about how it was pronounced. In the end, I simply accepted the spelling that was on my birth certificate, as this seemed easier for everyone.

Ruth, was a bit of an odd character. She lived with her mother and Nan in a large house on Queensbridge Road. She use to have strange turns. Once, in a music lesson, she put her head on the table as if she was sleeping, and when the pips went, everyone got up to move onto our next lesson except Ruth. I thought, "Here we go", and Janice and I rolled our eyeballs at each other. She was carrying on, and every time someone tapped her to move, she aggressively shrugged them off. I was told to leave her alone and move onto my next lesson, while Miss O'Brien, the Deputy Head was called. Practically every student that was at that school dreaded Miss O'Brien. She had such a resonant, commanding and authoritative voice when she shouted. There was a similar event with Ruth after we had played rounders in the playground at lunchtime once. Miss O'Brien was called on this occasion too, and as soon as she arrived, Ruth came back to her senses. Ruth was such an attention seeker. We were due to go swimming once and in the lockers changing into our costumes, Ruth said she'd come on her period and so couldn't go. I thought she was just trying to get out of it, so I made her show me. She wasn't lying, that time. Every Christmas Ruth and I exchanged presents and she'd tell me what she got from her mum for Christmas, birthdays too, and every summer she went on holiday. She made my birthdays and Christmases seem as though they were lacking.

I started piano lesson more or less as soon as I got to Haggerston. So did Ruth. I remember telling her that I wanted my mum to buy me a piano. Months later she told me *her* mother had bought *her* a piano. It was the same thing with a sewing machine. I said I wanted one, next thing I heard was, Ruth *has* one. And that's the way it was between us it seemed. I wanted it, but Ruth got it. Her mother was only a doctor's receptionist, but it seemed as though she had a money tree growing in her back garden! My piano playing didn't go that well. I'd go to school early so that I could get some practice in, in the music practice rooms, and sometimes I'd practice at breaks and lunch times. But I just wasn't progressing. Whenever I attempted to play a piece of music, no matter how many times I'd practiced it, it was always punctuated with pauses where I was working out which fingers went where. So the music jerked along. It was *awful*.

Ruth and I played truant occasionally. Lunchtimes we'd go to the burger bar near Brick Lane, and take our time about coming back. We were caught once. We were really late, and thinking about what excuse we'd give to our form tutor, then Mrs Atkin. We were laughing as we were walking along the corridor to our classroom, and Mrs Atkin saw us. We didn't get into trouble, but *we* knew *she* knew we didn't have a legitimate excuse for being late.

P.E. was great but at that time, I really disliked swimming. The water was so cold, and I wasn't a strong swimmer. And then there was my hair. The water made it so coarse and brittle. Sometimes I'd go under the hair dryer afterward. It ended up feeling like wire wool. Anyway, in one session that we had, we'd been given instructions by the instructor and everyone else in my group had jumped or dived in, and were getting on with it. I, on the other hand, sat by the side of the pool, not wanting to get in. The instructor came over and said, "If you don't get in, I'll push you in." So I decided to brave the freezing cold water. As I slid in, my front teeth on my upper jaw hit the side of the pool and crumbled. I felt as though I'd put sand in my mouth. I swam over to our P.E. teacher (then Miss Topham) and showed her what happened. She laughed as she said, "Rosie what have you done to your pretty face?" When I looked in the mirror at my tooth, it looked as though I had a fang for an incisor where part of the tooth had chipped away. I went to the dentist with Ruth that afternoon, and the dentist simply cut the pointed bit off, and I thought it looked O.K.

We were put in detention in one of our P.E. sessions once. We had to sit in silence for a whole hour. Janice, Ruth and I got the book 'Wifey' out by Judy Blume, and sat through the session searching for and then reading all the sexual encounters mentioned in the book. Mrs Atkin had recommended Judy Blume as an author whose books we should read, but I don't think she meant 'Wifey'! I did a great deal of reading, but the books I read were mostly pulp fiction, Mills and Boons romances. Sometimes I'd spend the whole night awake trying to get through a novel that I started reading. I kept up my interest in netball, rounders and gymnastics. In rounders, Ruth and I made up a team of backstop and first base, and in netball I maintained my position of goal attack from primary school, and Karen Stone was goal shooter.

When I'd reached the age of 11yrs, I was allowed to attend
the youth centre at Daneford School, a secondary boys
school that my brother Payton attended during the daytime.
It was *fantastic*! There was so much to do. Lorraine S.
and I used to do dance classes together. A woman called
Violet ran them. We did tap, jazz and contemporary dance.
It was brilliant. She took us to the Pineapple Dance
Studios next to Covent Garden once. Simone came with
us. We did a jazz class and I couldn't help noticing during
the warm-up that Simone was much more supple than me
even though I'd been dancing longer. The youth centre also
took us sailing at the Banbury Sailing Centre on a reservoir
next to Lea Valley. When we were good enough, we were
allowed in a boat alone. On one occasion I operated the
main sail and Lorraine the jib. We had some trouble
getting the boat off, so I kept switching sides, trying to get
the wind to blow into the sail and then biff, the boom went
straight into my head. Lorraine just sat there in hysterics.
Great fun though when we did manage to control the boat.
The instructor allowed me to drive her speedboat once too.
That was even better. Back at the youth centre, we played
cricket and basketball and sometimes just hung out eating
sweets. We went horse riding on a couple of occasions,
but I wasn't much good at that. However I loved being
around the horses. They're such graceful animals and I
loved the malleability if their nose and mouths. We were
invited by a women's group somewhere in Limehouse next
to Mile End to watch a video once. They showed us
'Aliens' starring Sigourney Weaver.

My niece Dorothy, stayed over at our place frequently.
She started smoking when she was about 12 or 13yrs. I use
to smoke with her when we were out of everyone's sight.

She used to smoke during our breaks at school too, beneath the gym or by the bike sheds. Dorothy was in one of the lowest streams at school and she hung out with all the black girls that seemed a bit hardened and more stern. She was really extrovert. At home, we use to stuff tennis balls down our bras so that our boobs looked bigger. In the mornings on our way to school, we'd get an ice cream from the sweetshop, or a cream cake from the bakers for breakfast sometimes. Really nice!

I started my period *finally* when I was 13 years old. I went to the loo and saw a sepia coloured spot in my knickers and I thought to myself, "So this is what its like". A day later, I got mild stomach cramps and the flow of blood was heavier. In the early days, I wore my sanitary towel with the front end at the back and the back end (which was narrower) at the front. My pants got soiled, and it soaked through to my trousers. I had a party on my 13th birthday. On the spur of the moment, Claudia, Payton and myself decided to invite all of our friends round. We didn't have much to eat until my mum came home from work, but we blasted the music, and danced. When my mum got home from work, she had some food that we shared out to everyone, and half way through the party, I changed out of the dress I was wearing and put some scruffier clothes on, and went to the '*Ship*' park with Jane Baker (whose parents were from Barbados) and a few others. The '*Ship*' park was just across the road from where we lived and had a large concrete ship in it, some parallel bars and a concrete tunnel which always had urine and pooh in it. The parallel bars were great though, we did all sorts of acrobatics on them, and we'd devised many games that involved the use of the ship and the tunnel. Jane Baker's mum won the pools when I was 13, and Jane's whole family went back to Barbados to live. One day in Daneford School when it was closed during a holiday, we were playing 'had' on skates in the playground. Simone was 'on it' and she was bull chasing me. I slipped while trying to escape from her and broke my wrist. When I looked at my arm, I thought I'd faint it was so deformed. They took me to the hospital where my mum worked, *on skates*! I kept saying, "I'm gonna die, I'm gonna die", while crying. Payton said it happened to me because when he broke his leg a year earlier I put a jinx on myself by laughing at him. I had to stay in hospital overnight and I was in *agony* the whole night despite the pain killers I'd been given.

I use to pick my mum up from work sometimes. Sometimes, I'd help her out at her workplace washing the dishes in the kitchen and if I were hungry, I'd get a meal. There was so much *waste*. That's why my mum came home with heaps to eat most nights. There was a blackberry tree in the yard behind the kitchen in the hospital, and we would often in the summer pick the berries for pies. One winter, my mum and I were walking home from her workplace. It had been snowing, and the snow had turned to ice. I was walking along talking to my mum, and the next thing I knew, she was on the floor. I rushed over to her to find out whether she was alright and she looked up at me laughing. I laughed so much the rest of the way home, that I wet myself.

We had several dogs during this period (not all at once) and a black cat that followed my mum home one night, so we kept it. She called it 'Small Cat' except when she was calling it in at night when she called it 'Kit'. Whenever she called it, it came running home. Then one night, it just didn't come back. We thought perhaps it had found a mate, because we searched high and low for it, but we never found it. We adopted Claudia and David's dog 'Benji' too because he was so much for them to handle. I got home from school one day, and my mum said Benji had given her a lot of trouble that day. So I told him off. I got right up close to him and was shouting at him. He bit me, right on my upper lip. My lip spit open, and puffed up like a balloon. I had stitches in it, but it remained swollen for a couple of days. After getting the stitches, I thought, how am I supposed to go to school looking like this? One morning really early, Simone came knocking at our door saying, "Rosie, Benji's been run over." In my nightdress and nightgown I ran outside to the little park in the flats where she said he was. He was just lying there with his mouth open breathing heavily. I went to touch him but he snapped at me and then he stopped breathing, blood coming out of his mouth. I rushed home crying. Our neighbours wondered what the fuss was about and when I explained to her she phoned the RSPCA for us, as we didn't have a phone then. It took them forever to come, and when they did come, Benji was well and truly dead. As he was such a heavy dog, she dragged him all the way to her car.

My mum's mum died when I was about 13. I remember when my mum got the news, she went into my room, closed the door, and wrecked the place crying and screaming in tormented agony. I never got the opportunity to meet my grandparents as they were all in St. Lucia and were very old. Both my parents were the oldest children in their families, my dad being born in 1919 and my mum in 1925. It was when we were living at Firth House that I first remember my dad coming home drunk. He would pass through the flats where we were hanging out with our friends and stumble home. As soon as I saw him, I'd just run home and complain to my mum that he was embarrassing us. It didn't make any difference. At about this time my mum had a stroke. She was in hospital for months. I did the cooking sometimes and my dad did it other times. When she came home she had a physiotherapist come and see her to see how she was getting on, and when she saw how damp the flat was, she said it was time we moved flats. So she sorted it with the council and in next to no time we were moving again. My mum never fully recovered from her stroke. She regained agility in her face, but she walked with a limp permanently.

Chapter 4: Broke Walk

Regents Estate where we moved to was back in the
borough of Hackney. It was a brand new maisonette, and
we were the first ones to move in along our row. We had a
ground floor flat, but within the flat itself, there were two
floors. Don't ask me why they gave us a flat with stairs
when my mum just had a stroke, but they did. There was a
small garden that was divided by paving stones and steps
in front of the flat. My mum and dad occupied the main
bedroom upstairs and my brother Payton the room next to
theirs. My bedroom was the tiniest room downstairs,
opposite the kitchen.

At the end of my third year, I didn't get to choose all of the
subjects that I wanted for my 'O' levels for the next two
years. French which I really wanted to do fell in the same
'option' as music, and I wasn't going to forfeit music for
anything. Mrs Atkin, our form tutor at the time insisted
that we all choose at least one language in preparation for
the European Union. German was the only other language
on offer and it fell in the same 'option' as History, which I
really wanted to do, so I dropped History for German. I
really wanted to do Office Practice too but Mr Harris who
was our Head of Year, said I could learn to type in my own
time. He felt I should concentrate on *greater* things.

In the autumn term of 1981, in my first week back of my
fourth year, the whole year were gathered together in the
science lecture theatre waiting to be told which class they
would be in for Biology, and that's when I *saw* him. For

me it was a *coup de foudre*. Dr. Walker was a new biology teacher at our school who was also the Head of Science. He was tall, slim, had mousy brown hair and a deep voice. My niece Dorothy was sitting next to me at the time, and she was teasing me and pulling my hair not because she knew I fancied him, but because that was just her way. In the following years, I doted on and pined after Dr. Walker inwardly day after day. I wanted him *so* badly. I confided in my nieces Jessica and Dorothy every time I saw them. My sexual urges became stronger and stronger, such that I started to masturbate. I'd lock myself in my room or in the bathroom when I was having a bath, and masturbate my urge away. In biology lessons, I couldn't concentrate. I don't know *how* I passed the 'O' level. I was *profoundly* in love. There were a couple of trips away to Sayers Croft a nature reserve next to Shere in Surrey, run by a man called Mike Reed and his wife. It was during these trips that I sometimes intentionally found myself alone with Dr. Walker. I'd get up really early and go for walks, and what do you know, Dr. Walker happened to be going for a walk too. I don't think I was the only one who had feelings for Dr. Walker. Ruth also found herself alone with him on one or two occasions. As much as I wanted it too, *nothing* happened between us. Now and then I thought I caught him staring at me, but that was about it. I was terribly *self conscious*, particularly in his presence. When I returned home from our first trip to Sayer's Croft, I announced to my mum that I was a vegetarian. I stopped eating meat and fish completely. I didn't really have a reason. I saw a boy at Sayer's Croft who had his meals set apart for him because he was a vegetarian, so I thought I'd try. It was exciting and new. My eating habits see-sawed between binges when I'd eat my way through biscuits, chocolate bars and cakes, to eating tins of low calorie soup with a slice of bread. Dorothy was the same. We'd get together and console each other on our diets and how fat we were getting from binging and vow never to eat another chocolate bar or biscuit again. But we always did.

I did enjoy studying for my 'O' levels and C.S.E.'s though. I *loved* Maths, and in Child Development we had to spend a couple of hours a week, away at a nursery school. The children were so affectionate. In English, Mrs Atkin said to me (in a tutorial I think) that I wouldn't pass English, and indeed, I failed English Language the first time round. Music was also wonderful, partly because it was being run by Mr Sackman, but also because I simply *enjoyed* it. Once a fortnight, we had a trip to the Royal Festival Hall to hear classical music, *live*. In German, I had a German pen pal who came to London on holiday. As she was staying near Elephant and Castle, we met outside the swimming pool and I took her over to my place. We both loved chocolate so we ate some together and some Mr Kipling's cakes. We talked about exams. She said in Germany you only get three goes at sitting the same exam. If you don't pass it on the third go, that's tough!

As I progressed through the course of my 'O' levels and C.S.E.'s I saw less and less of Rosemary, Sharon and Lorraine. Most evenings, I had homework. The one parents evening I remember attending, was when I was accompanied by my sister Claudia. We saw Dr. Walker who fussed about getting another chair for us. My sister laughed at him because she thought he was such a 'fairy'. I told her I liked him and that he was really *nice*.

In the fifth year, I starred in the school production of 'Simplicia', a musical the script of which was written by Tony Purcell (one of the science technicians) and the music was by Mr Sackman. I didn't have a clue as to what it was about. I remember during rehearsals once, there was a ballet dancer called Susan practicing a ballet dance in her pointe ballet shoes with Mrs Diamond (formerly Miss Topham). She kept stopping and saying, "I can't do this", and then she'd start dancing again. She looked like the perfect ballet dancer wearing leotard and tights and a long ballet practice skirt. She looked *beautiful*. I'd never seen her around the school before, but Mr Sackman seemed to know her well.

My parents were the source of much embarrassment for me. My mum was more or less illiterate. Back in St Lucia, being the oldest child, she had to forego going to school to look after her younger siblings, so she never really had any schooling. The few words she could read she read by saying the name of each letter and then somehow arrived at what the word said. When I tried to teach her to read phonetically, she laughed at me saying it sounded silly. She was also overweight, had a high blood pressure and was diabetic. My dad on the other hand although never quite reaching the full status of a teacher, use to teach in St. Lucia. However, when he came to England, instead of continuing in that vein, settled for factory work because in the short term he could earn more money and he needed the money to pay for the fares of my mum and their children, and his brothers, to England. Anyway when my dad wasn't drunk, he was rowing with my mum over the bills and food. My mum told me that she never *loved* my dad. Her marriage was more or less arranged between her mother (my grandma), and my dad. In our flat itself, there was dog's hair everywhere and in the kitchen my mum was always slaving over steaming pots of something or other. I just felt as though it was so untidy and dirty all of the time, that I was ashamed to invite anyone home.

Meanwhile, Francesca moved to a bigger place in the city, Aldgate East and I often spent time there visiting. Terrence was having problems with his studies so we would tease each other, me calling him a 'der' brain, and him commenting on the size of my forehead. Gabriela, often complained to me about Justine, so I was forever being the mediator between them. My mum got me a piano, but it didn't make any difference to my piano playing. At about this time I got a job as an office cleaner with my sister Francesca. Every weekday I had to get up at the crack of dawn before school, and I cycled to Aldgate on my bike. Emptying the bins was worse. The office staff would have cups of drinking chocolate, not finish them and throw them in the bin. I thought it was *disgusting* so I packed it in after a few weeks. Then I got a job with Zetters Pools in Clerkenwell Road on Saturdays. The place was full of black girls all about my age and I didn't make one friend among them, and they chit chattered the whole day. Glady's Lavers (a black girl) who was in the sixth form at my school, worked in the post room at Zetters, away from everyone else. Just before she left, they offered me her position, which I took willingly. It was slightly better paid.

Chapter 5: Ups and Downs

The TV series Fame was televised in the UK in the early 80's. I was one of its captive audience, who fantasized about fame and fortune. Over the summer of 1983, Ruth, Janet and myself went to a summer Theatre School at the Curtain Theatre in Commercial Road. It was *amazing*! Everyone on the course was full of beans, really outgoing and chatty. I auditioned for the Music Theatre group and got in. What a nightmare that turned out to be. Everyone else was brilliant. They performed all the dance routines really well regardless of how difficult they were, and their voices were incredible. I on the other hand was fettered by a problem with practically every dance routine we did. The girls in the group were nice enough about it, helping me out in rehearsals and so forth, but it didn't do much for my self-esteem. Ruth and Janet on the other hand were having a whale of a time in the drama groups. After a few days I really began to regret auditioning for the Music Theatre Group. There was this *immaculate* looking drama teacher who looked as though she had just stepped off of the cover of *Vogue* magazine. She was blonde, taller than average, graceful and slender and always wore black. At the end of the summer school, she ran a drama class which Janet and I attended. She taught Alexander technique, we studied poetry and focussed on a play by Lorca, 'The House of Barnada Alba'. She asked my opinion about a poem we were studying once, and as in English classes, I was clueless. She retorted, "Come on Rosie, even my son has something to say about that!" Her son was 8 or 9 years old.

In addition to this drama class, I started going to the Weekend Arts College (WAC) in Kentish Town on Sundays. It was in particular for ethnic minority groups wanting to get into the performing arts, although the majority of people there, including the teachers were white. I took classes in singing, movement for actors, drama and jazz dance. In every class, I felt *out of it*, like I didn't gel with the others. Anyway, apart from sampling peanut butter and cheese sandwiches for the first time, I became friends with a black girl called Cecilia Noble. She wanted to be an actress and to go to drama school to do a degree. We had great fun together outside of classes. Waiting for the train to go home, we imitated Shakespeare or whatever play we were working on at the time. God knows where it all came from. Somewhere along the lines however, amidst all the excellence that was thrust at me in every class, I decided acting was not the career for me. Not long after I dropped out and lost touch with Cecilia. Something really scary happened to me one Sunday on my way to WAC. When I had become an adult according to London Transport and was eligible to pay adult fares, Ruth and I always tried to get out of it. Whenever we were travelling on the buses, we calculated our birth dates so that it seemed as though we were still children, and if an inspector came on the bus, we'd give our false birth dates. One Sunday I was on my way to WAC not having calculated the appropriate birth date, and paid the child fare. Would you *believe*, an inspector came on the bus. I showed him my ticket, and he asked me when my birthday was. I didn't know what to say. He stopped the bus at

Liverpool Street and threatened to call the police. Tears streaming down my face, I apologized for not being honest about my age. He took the adult fare off of me, and let me go. That really was a close call.

In the sixth form I felt really confused. University seemed like some distant institution that only middle and upper class white students went to. I certainly didn't consider it an option for myself, at that time. So in truth, there was no reason for me to stay on at school and do A levels, but the alternative (finding a job) seemed even less appealing. At least if I stayed on, I could continue seeing Dr. Walker, so that's what I did. I took Biology, History and Theatre Studies. My mind boggled in every subject particularly History and Theatre Studies which I hadn't preceded with 'O' Levels. In addition I had to retake 'O' level English Language, which in the sixth form was being held at Daneford School. In History we read through pages and pages of small print, which Miss Rackham would attempt to decipher by drivelling on afterward. In Theatre Studies we read plays some of the time which Miss Wilby commented on as we went along. I know I didn't understand any of it, but I felt as though she didn't either. I felt Dr. Walker wasn't that great a teacher too, but maybe my feelings about my A levels was simply a reflection of the general malaise I felt at this time.

There were three of us doing A level Biology, Trudy, Tania (both white British) and myself. Tania was from one of the lower streams in the 4th and 5th year, but I ended up becoming quite pally with her. Trudy had mousy brown hair and decided one day, she wanted to change it. She arranged to go to Vidal Sassoon in Central London to be a model for the day. She paid something like £10 to allow them to have their way with her hair. I was really intrigued, and told her I'd come to the appointment with her to see what they did. Now Trudy was a really quiet girl. She wasn't very outgoing. They died her hair blonde, gave her a perm with a quiff and told her to take care of it she was to gel it and scrunch dry it. It looked *awful*! The sixth form of our school was mixed with the sixth form of Daneford School, so for the first time in a secondary school setting us girls interacted with boys. Rhyss (from the Indian sub-continent), fancied me. He hung out with Michael Lavers (Gladys's brother whose parents were from one of the Caribbean Islands) who I really fancied. Michael however had his eyes on someone else, namely Kim Felton, a svelte white British girl.

In the first term of our A levels, Ruth had the bright idea that the sixth formers should put on a school production for Christmas. Janet, Debbie Mitchell, Ruth and myself were the main characters. Ruth had all the ideas. We did sketches from the St. Trinians, the Three Stooges and whatever else came from Ruth's dated showbiz interests. It was a pretty outstanding feat for a 16 year old though.

Dr. Walker took us out for a day during the course of our studying A level Biology. We three (Tania, Trudy, myself) and Dr. Walker bundled into his van and off we went to some remote country setting. Being shy, Tania and Trudy pushed me into the passengers seat at the front of the van. I was *so* self-conscious the whole time. Anyway, of what I can remember, it was a nice day out. Coming home, he dropped each one of us off at our homes. He left me until last which sent tremors up my spine, because I felt he did it to be alone with me. Just before the Easter holidays of our first year of A level (1984), he announced that he was leaving, but he gave us his address and said if we needed anything we could write to him. I was *devastated*! I wondered *how* I was going to go on without my weekly fix of Dr. Walker. Ruth kept in touch with him because she gave puppet shows as one of her pastimes, and Paul's sister hired Ruth for one of her children's birthdays.

During the summer of that year, Sai Fan, Trudy, Tania and myself went camping for a week. As usual my eating habits were beyond my control. I felt so *fat*, the others were so thin. I gorged on cakes biscuits and sweets, whatever I could lay my hands on that was sweet. Toward the end of our holiday I sent Dr. Walker a postcard. I didn't ask him any questions, as I didn't want him to feel he had to respond. A couple of weeks after the holiday, I got a letter from Perry (Dr. Walker) saying that he liked me very much and would like to see me. My heart skipped many beats. God, whom I spoke to most nights, had answered my prayers. In his letter he suggest that we go out to a restaurant for a meal, but being as self conscious as I was at that time, I thought it better if we go out for a day in the country, and that's what we did. We met in Ipswich, Suffolk, me having arrived there by train, and Perry by van, and we drove to quiet place. When he stopped driving, he said he had some wine in the back of the van, so we got out of the front seats and made our way to the back. He grabbed me in front of the van's back doors and kissed me. He thrust his tongue in my mouth, and when he'd finished kissing me said he'd been waiting to do that for a long time. I thought the kiss was *disgusting*, but didn't say anything. Anyway we got into the back of his van, and kissed more, while he groped my body. The more we did it, the more I enjoyed it. We drank wine, and in the beginning we were both lost for words. We walked in the forest close to where we had stopped and before we knew it, it was time to go home. We arranged to meet the following weekend at his place. He was 31 and I was 17.

At the beginning of the academic year, September '84, I dropped two of my A levels, History and Theatre Studies and started a new one, Psychology, which I was hoping to complete in a year. It wasn't being offered at our school, I had to go to City and Islington College to do it, which was then in Pitfield Street. I also took up 'O' level dance which was being held at the Barbican site of City and Islington College. My relationship with Perry occupied my mind full time. It was an obsession. In addition, the malaise I felt about my A levels didn't change. I just couldn't retain anything. Dance became my favourite subject. It was run by Rosemary Lehan who had only recently finished doing a degree at the Laban Centre adjacent to Goldsmiths College. Even though I wasn't very supple *still*, I was good at contemporary dance, and Rosemary encouraged me to apply to the Laban Centre. At about this time, I joined a band that Tania's brother was in called the 'Sacred Hearts'. I did backing vocals for them. It was an 'indie' band, not really the style of music that I liked. Along with my niece Dorothy, I also joined the Patient Participation Group which was run by our doctor's surgery. We both had the hots for one of the doctors, Dr Sam Heard who was Australian. I use to invent reasons to go and see him. Once, I went to him and said I eat too much sugar, and asked him what could be done about it. He laughed at me saying I didn't have to worry about that as I was not overweight. I went on the mini pill two weeks after I started seeing Perry Walker. I wasn't taking any chances.

Perry was a great cook. He lived in Yoakley Road, Stoke Newington. Whenever I went to see him, I'd starve myself the whole day so that I felt and looked slim when I was with him. It didn't help any, because whatever I ate, no matter how small, just seemed to blow my stomach up like a balloon. He also smoked, rolling his own tobacco, and after meals I'd copy sometimes although I didn't take it down into my lungs. We talked about school, the teachers, my friends and my family. I quizzed him about his past, in particular his previous relationship. He never quite gave a satisfactory answer as to why he and his previous girlfriend split up. They'd been together for 11 years, and he said she had changed. She got a new job working as a producer for Anglia TV. Prior to this she worked in a wine bar in Stoke Newington. She did her degree in English Literature. You couldn't get more different than Perry and myself if you tried. There were class, race and age differences between us. We spent a great deal of time in bed. I actually met Barbara in the flesh once. I came to Perry's place from work one Saturday feeling tired and a little shabby and there she was with him dressed in a black cat suit. She was very attractive. Long flowing blonde locks and an hour glass figure with voluptuous hips. She went upstairs and Perry slavishly followed her. I couldn't believe it, after all, he was supposed to have finished with her. She left shortly after. Half an hour after she left, I left too and stuffed myself on a packet of digestive biscuits with cream cheese when I got home.

I use to tell my mum that I was staying over at Tania's place in the early stages of my relationship with Perry. But one day she confronted me about it saying, "I know you've got a boyfriend." So I revealed all to her. Apart from the sidelong glances and hint of disapproval whenever I was getting ready to go and see Perry, she was pretty tolerant. Along with the clothes that came from her salesman friend at work, were nightdresses of various sorts. When I wore them at Perry's place, he laughed at me. Anyway in addition to what my mum got me, Tania and I scoured thrift shops and in particular Portobello Road Market on a Saturday morning.

During the Christmas week of '84, my mother had a party. I invited Perry along to meet my family. I was so nervous, but excited too. His presence made everyone reserved, except Terrence who was chatting away with him. He drank many shots of whisky that night, and when we danced together, he put his hands on my backside and pushed his groin against me in front of my whole family. I told him he was drunk and tried my best to make light of it. Toward the end of the night I asked my sister Claudia if she would drive him home. When we got to his place, late as it was, he wanted to invite us in for coffee, but I didn't think it was a good idea. When my sister and I got back home, the party *really* began for me. I dropped my reservations, Paul having left, and I danced and ate lots. The next day I couldn't believe my *ears*. I was upstairs watching TV and some of my brothers and sisters had gathered in the kitchen downstairs. They were discussing my relationship with Perry my brother Preston saying, "But she's so small," the adjunct being that he was so big. I *screamed* at them, I *mean*, who did they think they were prying into my business, and that more or less settled the matter. Perry was a hit with my mum. She *liked* him a lot. She cooked him a meal of chicken, dasheens, yams, and sweet potatoes with kidney beans which I took over to his place. I was sure there was going to be dog's hair in it. He could barely finish it, but said he enjoyed it.

Over the winter months in '84, I got a new job at Marks and Spencer, Marble Arch Store. It was Janice's idea. She said it paid better than Zetters. Don't ask me how she found that out. Anyway, we were each given a uniform, and it was wonderful in the beginning. The spread for staff lunches was *incredible* and at the end of each Saturday, they sold the food that they couldn't get rid of on the shop floor at a reduced rate to staff. I was placed in the men's socks department. Would you believe, I even had a visit from *Mrs Atkin* with her husband, just doing her shopping, she said. She also said something about hoping this wasn't going to be my career choice, and then left. Perry visited too, but said he hated Central London, and didn't stay long. A few weeks later, I was filling shelves in the men's socks department when I was called aside by one of the store managers. She called me into a store room, held the door open and shouted, "You stink! I want you to go upstairs take a shower and change your uniform." I couldn't *believe* it was happening. Totally and completely *humiliated*, I cried my way to the showers, took a shower and changed into a new uniform. I was too ashamed to face the friends I'd made in my department afterward. I went on a fast for the next three days.

Perry and I went away for weekends often. I think we went camping after the Marks and Spencer incident. I made a vegetable quiche and for the first time in a few days I ate something. We brought our bikes along. We had sex one night, and Perry made so much *noise*, I was sure the people in the next tent could hear us. The following morning when I went to have a wash in the washroom, there was a woman in there washing her things or *something*. I was desperate for a wash because I had semen in my underwear, I don't think we brought any tissues. There were no separate cubicles in the wash rooms and I just couldn't bring myself to wash my private parts in front of this woman, so I didn't. I stank so *badly* on the way home. As soon as we got back to Perry's place I had a much needed bath. We went to Yorkshire one weekend and stayed in a cottage. We were, more or less, the only people around for miles. It was beautiful, but the bed creaked like mad. We stayed at a house owned by some friends of his once. It was in Buxstead, Sussex and it needed renovation, but there were basic amenities. Once again we walked the picturesque British countryside. Perry came across some sea-kale which he said was very good for you, so picked some to take back. When we came across a sloe tree he in a zeal of excitement said they were good for sloe gin, so picked some of those too. After staying at this empty house for a few days, we went to stay with his friends that owned it, Phil and Martine. She was French and he was English. Perry flirted with her like *mad*. In the evening she said I was probably desperate for a bath after staying at her old house which didn't have any hot water. I wasn't, but I agreed with her anyway, and took a bath. At bed time she asked us if we wanted a double mattress or single ones. I giggled, I couldn't help myself. What a stupid question! Perry got upset, and snapped, "Single ones." That made me *really* angry, so I stopped talking to him for the rest of that day. We also went out for meals at a couple of restaurants, Indian, Turkish and vegetarian and at weekends we went swimming or played badminton.

Perry discovered a lump in one of my breasts relatively early on in our relationship. I went straight to my doctor who said it was probably a cyst. He also said getting a mammography would do more harm than good, so he advised me to keep an eye on it and to leave it be. If it grew larger, then I should go back to him and we'd take it from there. Luckily it did go away after a while. I also got thrush on several occasions. It was *awful*! Perry got it too a couple of times, so we went to the Genito-urinary Clinic at the Homerton Hospital to get it checked out. I asked the doctor what the cause of it was, and one of their answers was promiscuity. This added to my suspicions that Perry was cheating on me. But I must say, in the early days of our relationship, I almost *expected* him to be sleeping with other women. I felt I was too immature for him a lot of the time, and that he wasn't *fulfilled* in our relationship. I also started getting dandruff really badly in my teens. Perry noticed it at one point, and said it didn't bother him almost as if he knew I was worried it would.

There were a couple of trips with friends from school too. One with Tania away at her cousin Geraldine's who lived in Bournemouth. I also went with the A level English group, in the first year of A levels, to Stratford Upon Avon to see a Shakespearian play. In the guest house we stayed at we were provided with a full English breakfast which being vegetarian I couldn't eat, so I ate lots of toast instead. Someone commented on how little I ate saying, "poor

Rosie." Ruth butt in, "Poor little Rosie has only eaten *all* the toast!" She was right.

Before the night of my A level exams, I prayed to God solemnly asking him to allow me to pass them, regardless of the fact that I hardly did any revision. I told him, I needed them and that he knew that more than anyone else. I failed both of them miserably, and I got a C in 'O' level dance. I stopped eating for a couple of days and vowed never to speak to God again. I think Ruth was pretty much the only one out of all of us who passed her A levels. The others had to retake. I took Rosemary Lehan's advice and applied to the Laban Centre. I had to audition to get in. That involved participating in a ballet class, contemporary dance class, and having a physiotherapy examination. In the physio, they were looking to see how supple we were. The girls that I was with got their legs way up high in a *rond de jambe* and I barely got mine off of the floor. In the ballet class, I struggled, but in spite of my poor performance they offered me a place. I was *ecstatic*, because it meant that there was life for me after failing my A levels. Ruth got a place on a B.Ed course at Goldsmith's College, University of London.

I started wearing some of Perry's cast offs, as well as my sisters. I remember in the summer Perry while pottering about making bedside tables said he'd like to grow his hair long. I encouraged him to do it, but he commented, I wouldn't like him if he did. And sunning myself on the roof above the bathroom one day he said, "Not too dark. Don't stay in the sun too long."

Chapter 6: Operation Charlie

Going to the Laban Centre was a big mistake. In the
beginning I use to cycle there every day, all the way to
New Cross, thinking it would keep me fit. All it did was
build up a lot of muscular bulk on my legs and I was
advised by the physiotherapist to stop cycling after a while.
I was in the lowest stream for ballet. The ballet teacher in
the first term was ancient, at least 70, and still going
strong. In the second term we had Peter Curtis who was
also my tutor. There were classes in improvisation, several
classes in contemporary dance using different techniques,
folk dance and weight training. No matter how hard I tried
my hip joints just weren't giving. I was *stiff*! I felt like the
worse dancer in my year. My eating habits continued to
yo-yo between periods of binging, to days of near
starvation. Contrary to the stereotype about dancers and
their diets, I found the majority had a healthy relationship
to food. There were a couple that were extremely thin and
were still not eating very much, but on the whole everyone
had a good appetite, and ate. When I binged, I purged my
digestive system with laxatives so that I wouldn't gain
weight. There was a whole food shop just around the
corner from the Laban Centre and they always had a
supply of *fresh* nuts and raisins which I was always
nibbling on between classes. I use to see Ruth during our
breaks. As jolly as ever, having a whale of a time. I
became friends with a Dutch girl, Sarah Lindhart. She was
passionate about Art. She said she often went to the Tate
gallery and spent hours just looking at the pictures, saying
they were so *beautiful*. I think she liked mainly
Impressionist artists. I just nodded in agreement. She had

a room in a house, and invited me to stay over once. We ate lots of wholemeal bread and cheese. I told her that I enjoyed knitting and when she went to Holland she brought me back some black mohair (quite coarse mohair), that I made a beautiful roll neck jumper out of. She said wool was very cheap in Holland.

I went to Perry's place one evening and found he had a friend with him. Charlie. Charlie had ginger hair, and I think I recall him saying he was from Scotland, although he didn't have a Scottish accent. He didn't have anywhere to stay so he was staying with Perry. He was writing a book about his travels to some distant country which I'd only ever come across in an atlas. Most evenings they went to the pub and came back tipsy and I remember one night, Perry making a lot of noise when we were in bed together as if he wanted Charlie to know what we were doing. He was pleasant enough, but after a while Perry said that he wasn't happy about him being there so asked him to leave.

I stayed at Perry's often, even during the week when I had to go to the Laban Centre. Half way through my first class, semen would trickle down into my underwear, and soil my leotard. I felt as though *everyone* could smell me. But when I stayed at his place I listened to a lot of his music, but became attached to only a few. Joni Mitchell's the Hissing of Summer Lawn's and Blue, Joan Armatrading and some of the Eurythmics. Perry liked Van Morrison and got me one of his albums as a gift once. I made chocolate cake (which we had with strong black filtered coffee) with lashings of cream, jam and chocolate sauce over the top which sated both of our sweet tooth. At the weekends I went to the Queen Bee Modelling School. Nothing big. Set up by a black woman in a school hall for black youngsters wanting to get into modelling, but taught by a Turkish woman. Francesca told me about it. It was in Stoke Newington, so I'd leave Perry's place dressed up and in my heels, never mind that I was only 5'4". My body was rigid from the dance training that I had and I felt so pathetic trying to look and walk seductively, that I left after a short while. But the other black girls were younger than me, thin and not very attractive, and eating Mr Kipling's cakes said they wanted to go to the top.

Back at the Laban, life for me was tough, nothing like the TV series of Fame. No matter how hard I tried, I wasn't brilliant at dance, and I didn't have lots of friends. In the second term, the MA students used the first year Dance Theatre students (my year), for performances. We were divided into groups. In the group I was in, for part of the dance, I had to like a sheet of paper being blown by the wind, rise up on my tip toes, arch my back chest to the ceiling and arms spread out, and then contract into a turn and scurry off the stage. Each group had to perform their piece in front of the whole year and all of the teachers. I didn't know where to put my face after the following incident. In the middle of my performance, just as I was about to turn and scurry of the stage, I fell flat on my backside. Everyone laughed, and it simply reinforced my feelings about my ability. Marion North, the head of the Laban Centre applauded me afterward for being professional, that is, getting up and continuing with the dance. I struggled on for a few more weeks and then came to the crushing realization, that dance simply wasn't happening for me. I left on the 14th February 1986. I was 18 years old.

I had a meeting with Peter Curtis about my decision and all he seemed concerned about was the money that they might lose if I didn't complete the year. He arranged for me to meet Marion, the head, and she was the same. After much consternation, I wrote to the Education Department of Hackney who were paying for me to go to the Laban, and told them I'd quit and that they should stop my grant. Perry seemed really disappointed that I had stopped going to the Laban Centre, although he didn't say so, I could just tell. A month later, I went to his place while he was at work, and found a letter on the dining room table he was writing to another woman whom I gather he contacted through a dating agency. In it he described our relationship as 'odd and cloying' and it seemed the only relationship he cared for was the one he had with Barbara.

So I was unemployed for the first time since leaving school. I had a Saturday job at Ladbrokes which I got after leaving Marks and Spencer, but like the Marks and Spencer job, that ended unhappily. One Saturday when we were cashing up, the manager discovered that a pound coin was missing from one of the cash tills, and he wouldn't let anyone go until it was sorted out. He really made me feel as though I had taken it, so I didn't go back after that. A couple of days after my birthday in May I landed a full time job working with the Crown Prosecution Service (CPS) as a clerical officer. I was *ecstatic*! At the CPS we were divided into teams, and I was on the Stratford team with Maria Kearsey as my senior (an Executive Officer), on the support side. Her dad was a policeman, she went out with a black guy (which I gather her parents weren't happy about), and she lived in Essex. The solicitors or Crown Prosecutors on our team were headed by Clare and notable among them was Rob Saunders who was a proper English gentleman complete with bow tie. There was one black Crown Prosecutor, Michael Thoka, a South African who went to Cambridge University. Rob Saunders kept a stuffed gorilla on his desk and along with the other Crown Prosecutors, often came back tipsy after lunch and cracked jokes using his gorilla. The Head of the whole service was based at our branch of the CPS, and he gave me more attention than he did the other clerical officers. He once asked me how old he was. I didn't have a clue, but noted his grey hair, and said, "65?" He retorted, "48", and then abruptly walked off. Maria teased me about it afterward saying I'd upset him.

In the early days Maria walked all over me like I was a doormat. So much so that all of the other clerical officers noticed. She was an employee's worse nightmare. I got depressed about work and felt trapped. I came across a book by Anne Dickson, 'A Woman In Your Own Right', about assertiveness. I identified with the most passive character in the book 'Dulcie' and was determined to make a change. Shortly after, Maria in her usual way had put me down so that everyone on the team heard. I went to the toilets and *cried*. When I came out I asked her if I could have a word with her in the computing room. We went in and shut the door. I was really emotional but basically I told her we were both adults, and if she had something to say to me in future she would have to use a little more respect. *Well*, we became quite good friends after that. She told me a bit about her history, and we went to a dance class together at 'Bodywise' in Roman Road, and life generally improved for me at the CPS. A few months on, there was an addition to the staff at the CPS a Higher Executive Officer, Margaret Coles. When she was introduced to our team, she warmly said hello to everyone looking at each one in turn, but she never once looked at me. I decided then that I didn't like her.

I wanted to move away from my mum's place. I felt I couldn't invite friends round because the environment was always so chaotic what with the dog, my mum's steaming pots and my nieces and nephews, so I wrote a letter to the then East London Housing Association who were based in Stratford and surprisingly, they offered me a room in a shared flat that was in a tower block called Elliot Close. It was just across the road from work. It was so *exciting* moving into my own place. My brother Payton gave me a lift in his mini metro with all of my stuff and then he wished me well and left. I went into the kitchen which was joined to the living room, and the kitchen floor, which wasn't carpeted like the living room, was sticky. Tom came out of the first bedroom and I asked him what happened to the floor. He said he got pineapple all over it. I asked him if he was going to clean it up, and he said he would. Tom was going out with a black girl who was from Southampton. He wanted to be a taxi driver so was in the process of learning the 'knowledge'. Angie (white British like Tom) was a teacher who occupied the third room along. Her room was beautifully decorated. It was bright and colourful and gave me some ideas about decorating my room. Mine was the second room along that had a brown carpet. In all of the rooms, the brickwork was evident on the walls, and was painted white. I didn't spend a lot of money on decoration. Intermittently I painted some of the bricks yellow, and I got yellow and white curtains that let the light through. I got a cheap single bed, a metal shelf unit from Argos, designed for a garage, and Perry supplied me with a desk from his house. There was no need for a wardrobe or chest of drawers, because each room had a built in cupboard with a shelf at the top.

Back at work, there was a *great* girl called Edwina Simpson who was a vegan. She had spent a couple of years previously working in Sweden, and her boyfriend was Swedish although she herself was British. She said Sweden was *beautiful*. She was very thin, but hardworking and liked by everyone. We played badminton one weekend, and I thought I was good, but she was *brilliant*. Whereas I used my whole body to smash the shuttlecock and then, it never seemed to go over the net with force, she smashed it effortlessly and it sped across the net. She organised some trips away for us on WWOOFing weekends (i.e. Working Weekends On Organic Farms). We went on two weekend trips. For board and lodging you helped out on a farm or did whatever odd jobs they had for you to do. I think one of the farms we went to was in Essex, and the other in Sussex, but I could be wrong. The couple owning the Essex farm were quite young with two children, all vegan. On the Saturday morning, I came on my period unexpectedly, but I couldn't bring myself to ask the woman who owned the farm for any sanitary towels, so I made do with what I could find. There were some 'Lilets' in the bathroom, and I tried to use one of those, but it was painful inserting it, so I used heaps of tissue paper. The whole thing made me so nervous. In the evening, there was a barn dance which Edwina and I was obliged to go to. What a *nightmare*! I was asked to dance by a lecturer who was staying in a caravan on the farm. When we whirled around to the music, my skirts went up (not so that anyone could see my underwear), and the smell of blood infused my nostrils. I felt as though everyone at the dance could smell my blood. Anyway, the next morning I asked the guy I danced with if anything was wrong the previous night, and he said there wasn't. We had a short conversation during which I gathered he met with a group of people in a barn for '*Primal Scream Therapy*'. I was so relieved when it was time to go home. I was dying to be in the comfort of my own room. The Sussex farm was owned by an elderly couple. For breakfast one morning, we had porridge made with water which Edwina added *salt* to. Accustomed to sweet porridge made with milk, I asked for milk and sugar, and was given some sour milk and a little sugar. They condoned my disbelief by reminding me that sour milk was used to make yoghurt and cheese. They had a soiree on the Saturday evening at which I felt totally and completely lost. Everyone was white and middle class.

In August '86, I went to St Ives in Cornwall with some old school friends – Janet Lacey, Debbie Mitchell and Tania. We spent two weeks there and trekked and took bus rides around the whole of Cornwall. I had spent the past few months toying with the idea of re-sitting my A levels at evening class, and by the time the holiday in St Ives was over, I'd decided I was going to. I met this really good-looking boy at the CPS who was between college and University who said to me in disbelief, "You're not going to stay here for the rest of your life, are you?" While in St Ives, I'd decided that I didn't want to be at the CPS for the rest of my life. Tania had just completed a foundation year in Art at Camberwell College of Art, and got a place on a BA course at Farnham Art College in Surrey. Her life seemed so well mapped out and beautiful in comparison to mine. When I got back to the flat in Stratford I read a book I'd picked up at a book shop in St Ives, 'Fat is a Feminist Issue' by Susie Orbach. I read it in two days and immediately put it into practice. I discarded my plan of cutting sugar out of my diet, went to Sainsbury's and bought bags full of sweets, cakes and biscuits. I *ate*, and felt so disgusted with myself afterward that I threw everything that I'd just bought away. Over the next few months, I got in touch with the Women's Therapy Centre who ran sessions on compulsive eating, and joined a self-help compulsive eaters group. The group consisted of four of us in total – Debs, Jackie, Sue and me. We met weekly at each other's houses or flats and each week we analysed our way through our compulsive eating problem. Debs was fat, and in love with her lodger, Jackie was plump and going out with a black guy, and Sue ordinary sized like me was also going out with a black guy. They were all white British.

In September I enrolled for two A levels at Waltham Forest College at evening class. Biology and Psychology. In addition I got in touch with the Voluntary Workers Agency for the Borough of Newham and embarked on some voluntary work. They'd arranged for me to see an elderly lady who was agoraphobic and lonely, in her home. I went to her place on a few of occasions, bringing something to eat with me. In truth, we didn't have much to say to each other and after awhile, I became uncomfortable. Her flat smelled of stale milk but at least she had her wits about her.

There was a whole food shop just around the corner from
Elliot Close called 'The Whole Thing', which was funded
by a housing co-operative. I got to know the people that
ran the shop quite quickly. Perry suggested I introduce
myself and bake some quiches for them that they could
sell, so I did. There was Paul Riley, Cathy his partner and
Ricky, all white British. I stopped working for the CPS in
the spring of '87 so that I could concentrate on my A level
exams, and one day a week, I cooked for 'The Whole
Thing'. It was *murderous*, really hard work, and I wasn't
making any profit, I was just about breaking even. In
addition, they got fresh food delivered from a whole food
wholesaler, which was attractively packaged, cheap and
nice enough. So I thought enough was enough. I packed it
in after a couple of months. I became good friends with
Paul and Ricky though. As Paul lived a little further up
Romford Road, we saw each other often. We met for
breakfast occasionally and tea, all times of day. We
chatted about our relationships and everything. I loved
having tea at his place because he had a variety of flavours,
my favourite being vanilla and strawberry, and he used
Soya milk. Ricky was forever trying to sell me his
philosophy on life which entailed being infinitely
contented (nice enough), because worry he said was self
created. At the time I felt this was total egocentrism
because it meant forgetting about the needs of others and
cutting yourself off, but we had many long discussions
about it.

I failed Biology and got a D in Psychology, but that
summer, 1987, I went to France, Chancelade de Belair
deep in French countryside, alone. I pined for Perry and

imagined that somehow he was going to meet me there. France was *lovely*, apart from the insects. I was staying in a cottage that had been converted from a barn, and apart from the farmer that lived a few hundred yards beyond me, there was no one. I didn't venture far from where I was staying, there was no need. A travelling grocer came to the cottage a couple of times a week and I bought food from him. There was a really inviting garden attached to the cottage with tables and chairs and long flowing grass. I went to go in there one morning and saw a huge snake slither through the bushes. I kept away after that. My footwear was unsuitable. Not court shoes exactly, but lace ups with a bit of a heel. I had to buy a pair of plimsolls from Quinsac the nearby village, when I managed to venture out. The surrounding fields were crawling with crickets. The noise coming from them was so tremendous, that I never once walked in them. I tried going out for a walk in the woods a couple of times but was fettered by the flies buzzing about my ears and the thought of insects crawling on me. In fact my only acquaintance apart from the farmer who I said hello to when he was walking in the fields checking up on his cows, was his dog Sibel. She was really friendly and often stayed in the cottage with me. Not to say that the farmer and his family weren't friendly, but my inability to speak fluent French fettered communication with them. Apart from her, there was the radio that I managed to get onto a channel that played the audio lessons we had in French class at school. At night it was pitch black and I heard noises coming from the roof. I didn't sleep well in France. I was almost relieved when it was time to go home.

Meanwhile things weren't going too well for Terrence. Francesca went on holiday and left Terrence to stay with my mum. However he left my mum's place saying he needed something from home, and didn't come back. We went to Francesca's place in search of him, but as he had the keys, all we could do was call out to him. It looked as though no one was in anyway. The lights were out and everything was quiet. We informed the police. When Francesca got back she discovered Terrence had been in her house all along, with his then girlfriend, a Jamaican girl, Beverly who was about four years older than him. They slept in Francesca's bed and left it unmade, left clothes lying around the place, dishes in the sink and generally left the place in disarray. She got pregnant at about this time and gave birth to a daughter who Francesca adopted and called Bianca. Months later he also had gotten into some trouble with the police. He and some friends went to steal a video from a small shop. It would seem Terrence's role was initially to keep a look out in the getaway car but he ended up helping his friends to beat the shopkeeper up. He was arrested on attempted robbery and grievous bodily harm. A couple of months later he was detained for three months in a detention centre in Gloucester. My brother Payton and I went to see him. He seemed repentant although I can't say he was acrimonious at the time of the event. On the way back we went to Payton's girlfriends place. She lived in Swindon, was skinny, almost anorexic, Jamaican and her parents were quite well to do; they served as councillors or held some official local governmental position. Her name was Angela.

In June '87, I went back to the CPS as a temporary worker and met someone new. Cheryl Williams. My first impressions of her were that she looked really insecure, nervous, and kept her head down pulling her shoulders up close to her ears. She was one or two years older than me had blonde hair and a slight physique, and she went out of her way to befriend me. So eventually, we became good friends. She came to my place often after work and she chatted a lot. I discovered she was a member of the Labour Party and something like the Socialist Worker Party, and they often met in pubs for discussions. She also had three A levels in English Literature, Sociology and History and intended to go to University in October of that year. She was almost always late for work and subsequently got into trouble with management. However she was constantly praised by them, not so that *she* could hear them though. We were alone on the Stratford section one day, and she asked me what I thought about Margaret. I told her, I didn't like her. Would you believe Margaret came forward from behind the filing cabinets, and said something to us that told us that she had heard exactly what we said. I wanted the ground to swallow me up. I couldn't *believe* it. I was sure it was going to prejudice her against me *even more*. At my place Cheryl laughed about it and told me not to worry. Easy for her to say. At one stage, there was a national strike for civil service workers. There were no picket lines outside and everyone except Cheryl came into work. Once again, she was praised, Maria mentioning how clever she was. Outside of work, Cheryl and I went walking on Hampstead Heath and in Richmond, went to the cinema, to the theatre and we ate out. Two films that we went to see at that time were 'How to get ahead in advertising' and 'The Handmaid's Tale'. After seeing the latter Cheryl's comments were, "Men are Bastards," to which I agreed although I was entertaining my own ideas of what the movie was about. We were both perplexed by the former, at that time.

Cheryl asked me about Perry often, and she was dying to meet him, so much so that one day she actually did. They were both on there way to see me and arrived at the flat simultaneously, Cheryl so pleased she was unable to contain the laughter escaping from her, and Perry with a quizzed expression on his face when I answered the door. Cheryl and Perry talked about politics, Thatcherism being the prime topic. I listened. When she left Perry said to me, "I thought you said she was working class?" I responded, "Well she is, it's just that she has done A levels in the humanities." He was dissatisfied. Before she left to go to university Cheryl said that I should read the English literary classics in particular the ones that she had studied at A level English Literature – 'Wuthering Heights' by the Bronte's and she bought me a joint book of 'Lady Chatterley's Lover' and 'Sons and Lovers' by D.H. Lawrence. She said they were having a debate in the Labour Party once about black representation. She asked me whether I thought black people should have separate representation in the labour party? I didn't have a clue about the politics that needed to be considered.

As we had on many occasions previously, Perry and I split up. I don't recall what the reason for it was on this occasion, but a few weeks later one Saturday afternoon, I had just had a bath and washed my hair. I sat in my room in my bathrobe and a scarf on my head my hair underneath looking like a briar bush while I did some reading. There was a knock on my bedroom door, and I realizing who it was and seemingly embarrassed by the scarf on my head, whipped the scarf off of my head then soberly answered the door clutching my hair. Perry stood at the door and let out a huff shadows settling beneath his eyes, his mouth a solemn line as he took in my appearance. I was glad to see him but sorry he'd caught me with my hair uncombed. I mean, I'd washed my hair at his place before and he'd even seen me grease it, but that didn't stop me from feeling uneasy around him when my hair wasn't combed. I once asked him if he'd like me to wash his hair with the shampoo and conditioner I'd bought for my own hair from The Body Shop. He responded, "No chance!" Anyway I asked him to wait in the living room while I got changed. I quickly combed my hair into two plaits, which I tucked in and when I was ready, Perry suggested we go back to his place. In the time that we'd spent away from each other, I thought about our relationship a lot. The compulsive eaters group was bringing up a lot of issues for me and I made a list of everything I was unhappy about in our relationship. That night when I went to Perry's place, I took that list with me and we spent the whole evening me discussing the issues from my list and him listening. I felt fat. I probably had been eating slightly more than usual being away from Perry, but I felt clumsy too. He told me I had changed. We slept with each other that night and I went home the following morning. Later on in the day Perry called me to say it was best if we didn't see each other anymore.

In September I retook Biology A level for the third time, and also did Statistics A level. Between studying, I read the English literary classics. I got up at 5a.m. every morning and made notes on the previous day's lesson and nearer exam time I used the time to revise. I was devastated about not seeing Perry, and he was all I talked about at the compulsive eaters group for weeks. But I was determined to get through these A levels and go onto university. I'd decided that I wanted to be a Clinical Psychologist, so a few months later I got in touch with Goodmayes Psychiatric Hospital and did some voluntary work on an acute patient admission ward. I was really disillusioned with the treatment that I saw implemented there. It seemed the nurses were simply present to ensure that patients took their medication, which was prescribed several times a day. The staff nurse was an Irish man who seemed to find the whole thing amusing; he had a permanent smile on his face from which would escape the occasional titter when he was talking. The patients were from a cross section of the community. There was a young black male adult who even though he was strung out on medication still heard voices which were telling him to kill his father, and an elderly black woman who lived alone who said things just got on top of her and she had a breakdown. There was an elderly white man from the north called Hugh who was obsessed with knowing what day of the week it was. After you told him, a few minutes later he'd ask again and said he needed to know so that he could cash his giro. He was suffering from senile dementia. The hospital itself was in really beautiful grounds and I think it was built during the Victorian era. However the staff said it was soon to close down, as there was a move against this style of hospital with the governments new community care plan for psychiatric patients. In addition I popped into The Whole Thing every now and then, and had chats with Paul and Ricky. We philosophized for hours about the nature of consciousness or mind, transcendental psychology, Ricky's approach to life. I baby-sat for Paul and Cathy every now and then. Cathy had dread locks, and at one point I was shocked to discover from Paul one night that she was working as a prostitute, as she said she needed the money.

I had visits from the family every now and then. Terrence came by with his girlfriend, a white girl called Joanne. He said people kept staring at him in the streets, particularly black men. I told him to ignore them. I played him my Kate Bush cassette, which I first got as a gift from Tania, and he immediately latched on to Wuthering Heights, and wanted to hear it over and over again. Gabriela stayed over a couple of times and complained about Justine. I bumped into Nelson in Stratford who was doing a degree in Maths at Sussex University. I didn't think about keeping in contact then, but he would have been a useful ally and companion particularly when *I* went to University. Preston worked locally too, and lunchtimes sometimes I went to see him. Claudia was living in Bromley-by-Bow at that time with her husband Taylor. She got pregnant with her second child and was getting a bit depressed. So I took her to the Royal Festival Hall one lunchtime where we listened to live classical music, and we had lunch there too. It was great!

I had started practicing yoga at home. Gabriela bought me a couple of books; one on yoga and another on beauty treatments, so what with my vegetarian whole food diet which I justified with the explanation that it was healthier, yoga and the occasional beauty treatment I plunged myself full time into caring for my body. Most weekends I went swimming. When I wasn't doing that, I lounged around the flat in muslin kaftans that hung like a veil over my body, which my mum had gotten me, wrapping myself in a long cardigan whenever Tom came into the living room. I did a conditioning treatment on my hair once, which I got from one of those books Gabriela gave me. It basically entailed heating some oil, and when it had cooled, massaging it into your scalp and hair, and leaving it on for an hour or so before shampooing it out. When I did shampoo it out, my hair started breaking and falling out. I couldn't believe it! In between beauty treatments and healthy eating, I worked hard at my A levels and read a lot of fiction mainly. And then of course there was the compulsive eaters group who I continued to meet with once a week.

I loaned some books from Ricky, and pretty soon I'd decided I wanted to be 'enlightened' and have all the benefits that went with it. I meditated, sometimes attending the London Buddhist Centre in Roman Road for a free lunchtime session, and intellectualised my way into 'consciousness'. In May '88 on my birthday I received a huge bouquet of flowers from Perry. Well I immediately called him only to discover he was watching football with some friends. He told me how much he missed me and we arranged to meet the following week. We met in a pub in Islington. I was so happy to see him, and he me, so what followed next was beyond my comprehension. He said he'd met someone called Llanka a Czechoslovakian, she was pregnant and they were getting married. I couldn't help but notice the occasional giggle that escaped from his mouth as he told me and then in a spiel of words in the same breath, told me how much he loved me. It was unreal. I don't recall much of what took place after that, but I was devastated when we parted. Shortly after at home, I burnt all his letters in my room. They burnt a hole in the carpet, so I had to strip the floor of the carpet eventually. He called round a couple of days later. I was in alone and I didn't hide my anger from him. We sat in the living room in silence. I asked him what he wanted. He said he wanted me. In the armchair I was sitting in, I turned my back to him and looked out of the window. I cried and didn't even attempt speaking even though he asked me what the matter was. I thought I was going to spend the rest of my life with this man in spite of our quarrels, and now he was expecting a child with another woman, and planning to marry her. I wanted to kill him. I glanced round to look at him and caught what I thought was desire shrouding his countenance. I said in disbelief, "You want to sleep with me." He didn't deny it. I got up and he followed, catching my arm. I tried to pull my arm away, but in a grip belying his frame, he held my arm as if his hand were a vice and he simply stared at me, not saying anything. I told him he was hurting me so eventually he let me go and I went into my room. He followed. I got the bed ready and took my clothes off as he did. We had sex, me crying. Somehow, in spite of Perry's situation, we got back together. He married Llanka and we had an affair. He came to see me on the occasional afternoon, and I lusted after him daily.

I applied both to universities and polytechnics. I wanted to go to Bradford University in Yorkshire because at least I'd have a friend there. Bradford was the only university that offered me a conditional place on a BSc. in Psychology, and I was invited up for a day to take a look around the university. I stayed with Cheryl spending a few days there.

She'd had a perm put in her hair so that it hung in soft waves. When she picked me up at the station I thought she looked pretty stunning. Cheryl was doing a combined honours in the humanities. There was an African- Russian staying in one of the rooms in the same halls of residence as Cheryl. Cheryl said he was awful; he was lecherous chasing the girls in the discos. When I spoke to him, I felt really sorry for him. I felt it must have been really tough for a black person at university, which were mainly full of white people. Particularly when you went outside of London. There were a group of Christians who I overheard playing the guitar together and singing. I said they sounded really sweet, but Cheryl hated them. She felt Christians were always so happy. Cheryl also had a friend called Rebecca who she said was a real tart because she slept around. We had a really cheap meal at an Indian restaurant, which was nice and we walked the streets of Bradford. All the polytechnics I applied to were up north too except one. That was my last choice which was in Plymouth, Devon. Plymouth was the only polytechnic who offered me a conditional place too so it looked like it was going to be Bradford or Plymouth. A couple of weeks after I got back to London, I got a letter from Cheryl telling me that the African-Russian wanted to marry me. I was flattered.

I felt I couldn't have done better in my A level exams even if I tried. I learned everything back to front, and inside out. I was late for a Biology exam, and sitting on the bus on the way to the exam, I felt as though the bus driver was deliberately taking his time. I arrived in such a fluster that Mrs Thurstone quietly told me to calm down, and said that I had plenty of time. Cheryl got back from her first year at

Bradford around the time of my exams, and the night before one of my statistics exams, we stayed up eating and drinking and chatting. I didn't get a wink of sleep, but it didn't matter because I was really hyped up about the exam.

That summer I went back to the CPS as a temporary worker. I got a phone call from Margaret Coles who in addition to inviting me back to work announced that Noel Williams one of the Senior Crown Prosecutors had died. My first day back some of the black girls there confided in me about the racism they felt was endemic at the CPS. They said white girls that had started work there after them had been promoted when they themselves had remained in the same position. So I took it up with Richard, the Senior Executive Officer. I asked him what it meant to be an equal opportunities employer then I told him that the CPS was falling short of that. For everything I said, he had an answer and then he said, "Look my skin colour is more natural than yours….." I couldn't believe it. A slip of the tongue it may have been but it *did* reveal his thought patterns. Anyway, the next day they moved me from the Stratford team where I usually sat, and put me to sit on a table all alone. I asked Maria if I'd done anything wrong, and why I was made to sit on a table alone. She said nothing was the matter. I became quite nervous and paranoid, and felt as though everyone was talking about me. I took it up with the compulsive eaters group, explaining to them what happened at work, and they said I was right and that I shouldn't worry about it as I would soon be leaving to go onto university or polytechnic. I had applied for other jobs however and luckily I was successful with one of my applications. Another civil service post working for a national insurance contributions office. I was offered the job on a permanent basis. They didn't know I intended to go on to higher education in the autumn. I was training with a couple of other white British girls both of whom had sorry stories to tell. The one that was from the north and had come to London on promotion talked about victimisation in the civil service, and the other talked about sexism in her relationship with her boyfriend. Anyway, during a tea break one day, I was sitting on the section with the other workers, and a black guy came through the office with a tea trolley. They all started cracking jokes about him and laughing, and he was mumbling to himself. I feigned laughter, but the whole scene was unbelievable. Inside a little voice said to me that that would be me if I stayed with the civil service.

I left the compulsive eaters group shortly after. I felt I had had enough self help therapy and that it was time for me to act on what I'd learned. Apart from that I wasn't really eating compulsively anymore. My binges had settled down thankfully. In addition I decided that I would devote my time and attention to seeking God or enlightenment, and there was no place for therapy in this process. Angie, the teacher living in the flat moved out soon after and she was replaced by a girl called Lisa (white British) who Paul knew. He said something about her being bad news but didn't give any detail. She was dating a guy who rode a motorbike. She was quite coarse in character, and her movements were nervous. I was in the living room one morning quite early, and she came into the kitchen and said, "My boyfriends just left me." She looked as though she was taking it really harshly, so I attempted to placate her by saying, "Don't worry about it, men are awful," and then she went to her room. A couple of weeks later I was in my bedroom talking to Cheryl on the phone and I heard a window smash, then music playing really loudly each record being ripped from the player and replaced by another and furniture was being thrown about in Lisa's room. Cheryl heard the commotion on the other end of the phone. I locked my bedroom door while talking to Cheryl about what I should do. Lisa was having a nervous breakdown. She went into the bathroom and living room where she said, "Good. I've eaten all their f***ing cheeses." About 20 minutes later there was a knock at the front door and someone shouted out that it was the police. Terrified I'd bump into Lisa, I opened the front door where I saw a detective who I'd often seen in the offices of the CPS with a couple of policemen, and I pointed them to Lisa's room. They eventually coaxed her out where she looked at me black circles painted around her eyes and red lipstick painted wildly on her mouth and said, "I'm gonna get you Mitchell," and they took her away. There was blood in the bathroom with what looked like to me at that time without my glasses on, a foetus. I thought she had an abortion in the bathroom! Daljit came back not long after, I explained what had happened and we began the long process of cleaning up. What a day! I walked around for the next few weeks looking over my shoulders, thinking Lisa was going to pounce on me any minute.

On the way home from work one evening I bumped into Rhyss who use to fancy me at school. I asked him whether he still saw Michael, and he said Michael was at university studying Law. Rhyss sometimes worked as an interpreter for the Asian community in Tower Hamlets and he often spoke on the news for them. I saw him on TV one

evening. Anyway we arranged to go out for a meal. I
didn't invite him up to the flat because I thought he'd think
the food stains on the wall, which were caused by Lisa's
breakdown, were actually caused by me. So I looked out
for him from the window of the living room, and when I
saw him called down to him. We went into central
London, and I said it would be a good idea if we ate at
'Pizza Hut'. He ridiculed me saying, "You don't eat there
do you? That's cheap." So we went to a posh French
restaurant where he said he'd eaten many times before. He
quizzed me about politics and said that I was a Tory.
Regardless of my contradictions and my attempts to argue
my case as a labour supporter, he continued to insist that I
was a Tory. When the meal was over, he said he'd pay.
The waiter came over with the bill and Rhyss realized that
he didn't have enough money so I settled the balance.

Over the summer, Perry stayed with me. I saw him every
day after work and at weekends. We cooked sumptuous
meals and on a Sunday morning read the paper together.
He felt guilty about Llanka so went back to see her
occasionally. At this point Claudia had been evicted from
her flat due to rent arrears and was staying in my room at
my mum's place with Andy and Ashley her two sons.
Llanka called my mum and Claudia and told them I was
sleeping with her husband. They called me and asked what
was going on. In addition Anne, Perry's sister called me
and said, "Well I think Llanka is a great girl and the pair of
you are being little sh*ts!" I was lost for words, but I
called Perry and told him what had happened. That more
or less settled the matter between us. We decided that it
would be best if we didn't see each other anymore. Before

we parted he gave me a book as a gift titled 'Walden and Civil Disobedience' by Henry David Thoreau.

I met up with a few friends from school one evening. Janice, Lorraine, Cordelia, Ruth and Trudy. We went for a pizza in Bethnal Green. We talked about racism, and for once in her life Ruth seemed lost for words. Janice and I arranged to meet up for an anti-racist march that was being organized from Finsbury Park in Islington. This was at the time when Perry and I were together, and I asked him if he was going to come but he said that this was my shout.

The results to my A level examinations came through in August. I got a B in biology and a D in statistics, too few points to go to Bradford, but just enough to go to Plymouth. I called Bradford anyway to see whether I could coax them into accepting me with a B and a D as opposed to a B and a C which is what they were asking from me. The woman I spoke to looked at my application form, looked at where I lived and said, "Hackney? No definitely not, we cannot offer you a place," and that was that. So I was set to go to Plymouth. When I called Paul to tell him about my results, he was with a group of friends and as he picked up the phone I heard he was talking about me to them, saying something about my being paranoid. Subsequently I distanced myself from him a bit, but we remained friends, after all, I didn't have that many friends. Before I went to Plymouth Perry warned me about it saying, "Why don't you stay in London, at least there are more black people in London," but I was all set to go. I wanted to leave London and start afresh somewhere else.

Back at the flat I was in the kitchen one evening alone and I got a terrifically sharp shooting pain through my bowel. I immediately drank heaps of water and the pain subsided as quickly as it came, but it was frightening. I was in the living room a little while after when Lisa came back into the flat. She was on medication and shaking a little. She had been in Goodmayes Psychiatric Hospital but I had stopped doing voluntary work for them by that time. We had a short conversation during which it seemed she couldn't remember any of what had taken place last time she was at the flat. I got ready to move to Plymouth.

Chapter 7: Off to Polytechnic South West in Plymouth

In September '88 I went to Plymouth for the day in search of accommodation. I had rejected a place in halls of residence. I decided being 21 years old, I didn't want to be around lots of screaming 18 year olds. When I arrived at Plymouth station I got wolf whistles from two white boys so I thought Plymouth can't be bad if they're wolf whistling black girls. I went to the accommodation office and got a list of three addresses that I was to check out. I bumped into a woman who I believe worked for the church and she asked me what I was doing in Plymouth. I explained I was soon to be a student at the polytechnic and I was looking for accommodation. She said she knew of an African woman who had a room in a council flat. She had a couple of kids, but she implied I'd feel at home there. I said thanks but no thanks. I didn't come all the way to Plymouth to be stuck in a council flat. The first house I checked out was an absolute dump. The furniture was of a poor quality and the flooring was awful. I thought I'd never feel comfortable studying here so I moved on to the next on the list. The next house was in a place called Stoke, in Napier Terrace. It was owned by Gregory and Jackie Yates who had two children between the ages of 5 and 8 years old. It was a really nice house, so if it was OK with them, it was alright with me. Jackie was a housewife, and Greg was a solicitor. They had a French girl staying with them too who was working as an assistant in a nearby school. Jackie said the only thing required of her lodgers was that they baby-sit occasionally. I thought that was fair enough, so I was all set to come to Plymouth. I asked her if it was OK if I had friends stay over some weekends, and she said that that was fine.

Back at home, I got things ready to go to Plymouth. I moved all of my furniture back to my mums place. My period was late and I kept having strange stirrings in my abdomen. I was really sorry to leave Elliot Close, it held so many important memories for me. I got a lift to Plymouth from Paul with my things, and I was sick on the way there.

Of the psychology freshers, I was the only black student. During our first meeting together it was as if everyone knew each other there was a hubbub of conversation. We were given a pep talk by the chair of the polytechnic during which he emphasized the social aspect of being in a higher education establishment, saying that we should all be *mixing* with each other. We were given some forms to fill in about our backgrounds e.g. parent's occupation, A level results etc. etc. by a female lecturer. I was sitting next to a mature student called Veronica at that time who seemed very interested in what I wrote on my form much to the disapproval of the lecturer leading the session. We were divided into groups and shown around the polytechnic. It was during this time that I met Rachel Buxey who stood out for me because she seemed to have a spiritual aura about her. She said that she *was* into spirituality as it happened. We didn't talk much at that time.

During one of the first few days at the polytechnic, there was a pub-crawl for psychology freshers that began at the students union. Accustomed to my chats with Cheryl about the plight of the working classes, I assumed that all the students were *from* the working classes. I was disappointed to find that that was not the case. Anyway, I ended up in a pub with a fat girl called Cat (short for Catherine). I thought I'd be safe with her because at least we'd have compulsive eating in common. We were joined by a ginger haired boy called Steve Russ who I at first thought was awful he was so full of insecurities *and* talked about them. Back at the Yates' place I met Isabel the French assistant who seemed really nice. She was here learning English ready for the European Union she said. We went to a pub one night and bumped into some of the students from the psychology course Steve included. In spite of my trying to make conversation with him, all I remember was him looking at her long slender legs which were on display due to a knee length skirt she was wearing that night. I went to Dartmoor one Sunday with the Yates' and there two children. We visited an old church in Bretnor which was high up on a hill and had really beautiful views, and a castle in Lyndon. We had tea in a teashop, and I must say I felt self-conscious enough without having Alexander the younger of the two children saying to me, "Why have you got such a big nose?" My reasoning failed me at that time, and I was just plain angry.

I was sitting alone during one of the lectures when a couple of Indian girls introduced themselves to me, Nisha and Meenaxi, both Hindu's. They said if I wasn't hanging out with anyone that I could hang out with them. I thought that was really nice of them, and from that point on, they became my pals. My period still hadn't come, so accustomed to getting pregnancy tests done by my doctor Sam Heard in London, I went to see the polytechnic doctor. He was completely unsympathetic saying abortions aren't the nicest things for doctors to have to carry out and told me I'd have to get a pregnancy test done at a chemist. So one lunchtime at Woolworth's having tea and cakes with Nisha, Meenaxi, Man Yee (from Hong Kong), Gemma and Jane (both white British), I excused myself telling them I'd be back shortly and went to the chemist to get a pregnancy test done. My fears were confirmed. I was pregnant. When I left the chemist my mind started spinning literally as I wondered what I was going to do next. Back at Woolworth's I told them I had a rash on my back and I went to the chemist to get some ointment for it. When I got back to the Yates' place I flicked through a diary I had picked up at the Women's Therapy Centre that contained lists of useful phone numbers for women and I called a private abortion clinic in London. They made me an appointment for a consultation the following week. My eating habits were beyond my control. I had gone off of whole foods and was eating chips most nights and ready cooked meals that I had only to pop in the oven. Every morning I felt sick unless I ate something. My breasts enlarged and were secreting milk, and it was really painful attempting to empty my bowel in the morning and when I did, hardly anything came out. Desperate for someone to talk to about it all I called Perry. Greg and Jackie were listening in the kitchen to my conversation so I simply repeated on the phone, "I *need* to *see* you," and he soon caught on that I was pregnant and came to Plymouth the next day. I told him that I intended to get an abortion and he angrily retorted that it was all just like plucking off a toenail to me. He also said, "I might want it," but I had already made up my mind about the abortion.

I met Perry at the station when I went for the consultation. He came with me, not to the actual appointment, but to the offices where the consultation was to take place in central London. The examination showed that I was approximately two months pregnant, and they fixed me an appointment for the abortion at a clinic in Richmond the following week. Perry and I went to a pub just across the road afterward. He was upset and threw £350 cash at me across the table saying that was all the bank would let him have in cash at the moment.

The following week when I booked into the clinic I was sharing a room with a girl who was also a student from Luton, studying physiotherapy. She was really pleasant. The clinic looked like a guesthouse that was in a quiet street. I was given a general anaesthetic for the operation and when I came to it was as if nothing had happened. The same evening, a woman came round with a trolley full of sweets, some of which I bought. In the morning, breakfast was provided for us, and then we were allowed to leave. I was really happy when it was over with. I thought now I can finally concentrate on studying. So I was really surprised and angry when I arrived at Paddington station to see Perry waiting there for me. I couldn't believe it, after all he had a wife and child back at home and we both already made it clear that nothing could become of our relationship. He got on the train with me, and in spite of my efforts to ensure that we didn't talk or that he didn't sit next to me, he sat next to me. Soon after that he was kissing me and telling me that we could be together. I relented. We stopped off at Reading so that he could go into work to clear something up, and then we made our way on to Plymouth, but got off a few stops early and went to an inn to have some lunch. He said he'd come to see me at the weekend.

In the evening Isabelle had a friend over from France, Giselle. They were talking in the kitchen and Isabelle was laughing at her friend because her parents were farmers who lived in the countryside and were relatively poor. I kept my mouth shut. Along with Isabelle's brother, they'd arranged to go to Totnes the following day which was a couple of stops away from Plymouth and I was asked if I'd like to go with them to which I'd said I would. So the following day saw us in Totnes. It was beautiful. It was a small place more like a village than a town, and quaint. It was full of whole food shops, thrift shops, craft shops and there was a really colourful feel to the place. There were some castle ruins there too which we visited. So we wandered up and down the main street in Totnes, popping in and out of the shops until it was time to go home.

The Yates' house was freezing, particularly during the daytime when Jackie was in alone and decided not to have the heating on. So during free periods when I was suppose to be studying, I'd go back to my room at the Yates place and try to study, but found it impossible because it was so cold. I bought an electric heater eventually which must have made the Yates' fume if they had the heating off in the daytime to save money, but I was beyond caring. I had invited both Tim and Rachel over on different occasions, both first year psychology students. Tim was a vegan, Rachel a vegetarian. With Tim I talked about spirituality and got him to listen to my cassette of western spiritual guru Da Free John speaking. Rachel was much more intense and personal, so I ended up telling her my life story, including details of the recently carried out abortion, over a meal of vegetarian shepherd's pie. Apart from being a latter-day hippy she was also a feminist. We were discussing an essay that we had to write about women's oppression once to which I casually said that you could write anything for that. She yelled something like, "It's *true*! It's not about writing anything." But we became quite good friends anyway. A few months later, Rachel told me that she was pregnant and that it was no big deal, but she was having an abortion. I cried when I heard, apologizing to her. Somehow I thought it was her connection to me that had caused the pregnancy and impending abortion. There was a student march organized in central London which I attended. It was against student loans. I went along with Tim and a few others from the psychology course. Coaches were provided for us by the union. There were thousands of students, it was really well attended, but it didn't stop the government from bringing in student loans in the '90's.

At the weekend following the abortion, Perry and I went to Cornwall. He brought his car, so we just drove around until we came to a quiet place where there were a couple of cottages and he asked if they had a cottage free for rent for the weekend which they did, so we stayed there. We walked the Cornish countryside and the woods nearby. Breakfast was provided for us by the landlady and we went to an inn for something to eat in the evening. Back in Stoke, Devon, I began searching for a place for Perry and myself to live. Things were becoming quite tense at the Yates' dwelling. One evening they asked me if I would like to watch a video with them. I consented, to find that the video was called 'White Mischief'. I don't recall what it was about now, but the title spoke volumes. Anyway, sometime in November, Perry and I found a place to live not far from the polytechnic in Restormel Terrace. It was a house that had been divided into two flats. There were a couple living in the upstairs flat and we occupied the ground floor flat. It had two bedrooms which we made into a bedroom and a living room, and a dining room and there was a small back yard in which you could hang washing. To gain access to this, the couple upstairs had to walk through our dining room and kitchen. So Perry stayed in Reading during the week, and in Plymouth at weekends. It wasn't easy. I'm sure he felt guilty about having left his wife and child, and staying in a flat in Reading alone couldn't have been pleasant, but the whole situation was of his own making. I placed no demands on him whatsoever. Before I left the Yates' place I left a note in Isabelle's room with my address on it telling her to come and visit. She didn't once come and visit me. I think the note was confiscated by the Yates' before she got to it.

I became Pals with a second year engineering student called David who I met at a contemporary dance class at a community centre in the Barbican of Plymouth. He had a really big nose just like the actor Karl Malden from the Streets of San Francisco, but was a really nice guy. We had similar tastes in music and he played the guitar like me, although he was much better. I also did classes in yoga in which I realized I was still not very supple even though I'd been practicing it for some time and I joined the community action team in which along with a girl called Sue I did some voluntary work at a day centre for the Royal National Institute for the Blind. Here I felt I wasn't received as readily as was Sue by the other workers and the users of the centre, some of whom were partially sighted.

The next time I got my period was at the weekend when Perry was present. The foetus which I thought had been extracted during the abortion, came out after some strong period pains. I went to the toilet, and there it was. I was hysterical and ran to Perry explaining what had happened. He more or less told me to stop being so melodramatic. He was completely unsympathetic. Contraception was a problem for me too. On the mini pill I always got thrush. Perry didn't like using the sheath because he said it interfered with his feelings during sexual intercourse. I would never consider using the I.U.D., so the only other option left to me was the diaphragm. I had to go for a fitting of the diaphragm, and it proved very difficult to insert. Not only that, although I wasn't small, I wasn't exactly large either, and the nurse said I needed the largest size out of three sizes that there were. Rachel had a diaphragm, she was fatter than me and had the small or medium sized one. During sexual intercourse, Perry complained about it, saying he could feel it, and that he really didn't think it was a good idea. So I stopped using it. Anyway a couple of weeks before Christmas of that year Perry and I were having an argument about something or other. We were in the dining room when he said something mimicking a Jamaican accent simultaneously. I just walked away and didn't bother rising to the bait. Hours later I went to the bathroom, and when I got back into the living room found a letter from Perry explaining briefly that he had gone back home for good. I busied myself with rearranging the flat into two bedrooms again and thought about the heaps of work that I had to catch up on. I spent Christmas of 1988 alone.

At the beginning of the spring term in January '89, I announced that I had a room to let in my flat. Meenaxi said she was unhappy with her accommodation and was looking for somewhere to live, so I showed her the spare room at the flat. She was happy with it so shortly after moved in. It was really nice living with another female doing the same course. We went to lectures and shopping together.

I don't know what it was, but during lectures or tutorials, whenever I had the opportunity to speak up in class, I became filled with a crippling anxiety and got extremely nervous, so I never said anything. I remember in a Developmental Psychology lecture, Dave Rose the lecturer (and my tutor) talking about child abuse. He said often the memories were so painful for the victims that they blotted them out and were left with an anxious disposition. So I got it into my head that I had been sexually abused by my father, and the experience was so painful, that I had forgotten it. I thought that was the reason that I experienced so much anxiety. When I got the opportunity, I bought books on child abuse, and worked through the exercises they suggested and treated my father suspiciously whenever I was around him. But never once did I recover a memory about being sexually abused.

There were a couple of black girls that I saw together around the poly often, and whenever I passed them, they were always laughing. I thought I'd better introduce myself to them, so I did. The fat girl was called Faith and was studying biology, and the smaller girl was called Yvette and was doing a social science degree. They were both from London and as far as I was aware had parents who were from one of the Caribbean islands. Faith was really talkative, and she took it upon herself to start up an African-Caribbean Society, the first of its kind in the poly. She approached me about it one afternoon, as she did all of the African-Caribbean students around the poly, asking me if I'd be interested. She needed to have a certain number of people interested in order to be able to start up the society. I thought it was a great idea. The opportunity to meet similar others was mind blowing for me at that time. At our first meeting everyone was really excited. There weren't many women admittedly, but everyone was feeling the effects of icy cold Britain surrounded by white people. People were cracking jokes and everyone was in good spirits. When it was time to vote in the chair of the society, I thought the obvious choice would have been Faith. Not so, however. I was voted in as chair. Don't ask me why. I didn't say much. I immediately became filled with anxiety and realized that I was truly not qualified to lead the African-Caribbean Society. All of my knowledge about the history of black people had come from the movie 'Roots' which I saw when I was in my teens. I knew nothing else. So I declined the offer of chair saying that Faith was better qualified than myself and became vice chair instead. At the end of the meeting, I invited everyone back to my place for tea and coffee. People made jokes that the white people would think that there was going to be a riot at seeing so many black people together in one place in Plymouth. Anyway Meenaxi was in when we got to my place, and she helped me make tea and coffee for everyone. For a few hours we sat around chatting and laughing. When they all left, Meenaxi asked me if she could join the African-Caribbean society as it seemed like fun. I told her I'd ask Faith thinking nothing of the fact that she was Indian. I asked Faith, who after a few moments of deliberation consented.

Friday evenings we strutted our stuff at the Rizzy nightclub along with all the other students from the polytechnic. We had a wild time back then. Faith came to our place occasionally during her free periods and study days, and it was on one of these occasions that fool that I was, I confided in her about my anxiety. I also told her about the relationship I had previously with Perry. She laughed at my experience of anxiety and used it against me in African-Caribbean society meetings. You see, Faith liked a guy in the African-Caribbean society who happened to like me, and I believe this amongst other things perhaps, was the reason for her resentment towards me. She told me she was a member of the Windsor Fellowship which was a scheme set up in South London where she lived that mentored young people from the ethnic minority community in an attempt to draw them into higher ranking positions in the Civil Service. Richard, also a member of the African-Caribbean society, liked me lots. He was really handsome, but all the other guys found him amusing. At that time, that put me off of him, but I now realize it was probably just envy on their part. In addition I was shamelessly chasing white boys. I was infatuated by Steve who became more appealing to me by the day. He was clever, good looking and unlike what I felt about Richard, I decided he was 'deep'.

Richard and I became quite good friends. He plied me with complements and told me he even slept with the bank manager of a bank in Plymouth he was so desperate. At a party Faith gave one day, I noticed the white girls throwing themselves at him and told him he didn't have any problems whatsoever. I ditched the party to pay Steve a visit who had previously said I was welcome at his place anytime. He was living in halls at that time, a tower block adjacent to the poly. When I got to his place I found he was in the kitchen with another girl from our course and another couple. She immediately left when she saw me, and Steve looked uncomfortable. I asked if I was interrupting anything to which he said I wasn't and then proceeded to get his shoes on so that we could go out for a walk. He had a poster of the singer Sade on his bedroom wall, and said he was a great fan. The walk didn't amount to much. We went to the Hoe by the sea, and came back again. My infatuation grew.

I invited Steve round to my place once. We ate, listened to Joan Armatrading and talked a great deal. At the end of the evening, he said he had had an unforgettable experience. And that was all. There was no indication that we could be an item. I think he had a girlfriend in London anyway, although he himself was from Swindon.

Once a week Meenaxi and I played badminton, and there I came across another swell looking white boy called Matthew DaRosa. He wolf whistled at my badminton playing which made me think maybe he was interested. However the same night on the way home in the van he stared unwaveringly at Meenaxi. I decided this was because he thought I was overly ostentatious in badminton and was shying away. When we got home, I asked Meenaxi what she thought of him. She said she thought he was ok but she didn't fancy him which I thought was just as well. In the evenings we often went to the theatre, cinema and in our days off we sat by the sea on the Hoe. My dandruff was still a big problem for me, and I often confided in Meenaxi about it who said she had similar concerns. She talked about it being difficult to get rid of, and it getting stuck in her hair which was extremely long, but then she was Indian.

During the Easter holidays, I stayed in Plymouth in order to catch up on some much needed work. I had a visit from the police. A detective and police officer came round to my place and invited me for an interview at the station. They said it concerned an Access card that was issued in my name. When I went to the police station, two officers interviewed me, and just as seen in programmes about the police, they recorded the interview. They then proceeded to interrogate me about the Access card. It seemed someone had opened an account in my name, forged my signature and spent just over £1000 on clothes and in restaurants. They accused me of being a desperate student who was stuck for cash and couldn't resist the temptation of spending the money available through an Access card. Their accusations came hard and fast, and I really thought I was going to be charged for something I hadn't done. It was frightening to say the least.

At one of the African-Caribbean Society meetings Faith announced that we would be going to see a movie by a new black director Spike Lee, called 'Do The Right thing'. I'd never heard of him before, but most of the others had. It was shown at an Arts Centre in the Barbican in the summer term of '89 and a whole load of us from the African-Caribbean society trekked along to see it. The movie was a feast for my eyes. I fell in love with Spike Lee there and then and decided I was going to marry him, never mind that he was a movie star and director. I'd never seen anything like it before. It was so fresh and artistic and I felt all of the characters no matter how lowly they were, were animated, and everything seemed so clear. I also got an education while watching it. The following week at the African-Caribbean society I led a discussion on the movie as Faith was away. Luckily for me a Nigerian girl called Janet Ogendengbe came along who talked a dozen words to the second, and she was *loud*, so that the discussion didn't dry up as I feared it would. Janet O. was to become a useful ally to me later on, although at first I shied away from her extroversion. A little while after things became quite tense between Faith and myself, Meenaxi being our neutral ground. Eventually she angrily accused me of leaving all of the work to her at a meeting one evening. The anxiety rose up and stuck in my throat, and I couldn't answer, so I stopped going to meetings, and stopped talking to Faith. She still came round to our place, but this time only to see Meenaxi who had become the treasurer of the African-Caribbean soc.

Richard and I went to see the movie 'Mississippi Burning' once I'd left the African-Caribbean society. We were the only black people in the audience. I was pretty frightened and joked that we'd probably be lynched once we left the cinema. Richard on the other hand was excited, and found it all amusing. I couldn't understand why.

Meenaxi's tutor was Dave Stephenson who was also the lecturer on Behaviourism. Throughout the first year in behavioural psychology lectures we had a series of worksheets to work through a percentage of which we had to pass to go through to the second year. I didn't sweat over them, but I worked hard enough and even so I was one of only two people who failed. I couldn't believe it. Anyway it meant I had to go and see Dave Stephenson who was a bit of a mystery man, but that made him all the more appealing like most of the male lecturers, not that they were all as mysterious. Something about age and knowledge that makes men extremely attractive when you're a student. Meenaxi on the other hand said she didn't like him at all. I had to do an essay for behavioural psychology, and with that I was through to the next year.

A conference was held every year for final year psychology students to present their final year projects, an experiment or study, that they'd worked on during that year. All psychology students were invited to attend either to present projects, or to observe. In my first year it was held in Bristol polytechnic and Meenaxi, Nisha, Man Yee, Gemma and myself decided we would attend. We went by coach and were accompanied by Steve Newstead then the Head of the Psychology Department and Ian Dennis the Head of the first year. It was a pretty strange day. I was self conscious the whole time and Nisha didn't help, laughing at my shoes. Apart from being ushered along to presentation after presentation I received a great deal of attention from one of the lecturers from Bristol who was at least in his 50's, although I didn't feel it was sexual in nature. At lunch time we were provided with lots of fresh fruit, cheese, French bread, crisps and fruit juices and as I was trying out veganism at that time, I had a banana and potato crisp French stick. At the end of the presentations we were given the opportunity to speak to the students who gave presentations and the Plymouth crowd announced that they were going to a pub with the lecturers. Meenaxi et al including myself didn't want to go, so they left it to me to tell the lecturers. Wrought with nerves I spoke to Ian Dennis who with an extremely concerned look on his face told us when the coach was leaving and that we should meet them at the coach. Meenaxi & co. and myself went to the red light district where we had tea and coffee in a café.

Around the time of our first year exams, Man Yee and myself went walking in the Barbican, and came across a holistic health centre called 'The Rainbow Centre'. When we arrived there they were in the middle of having a meeting on spirituality which I gather they had every week. There were various dishes of food placed on a mat to one side of the room, and everyone sat around listening to the speaker. I felt really at home there, and we were invited to participate. I received a great deal of attention from the speaker who I later learned was a Moslem called David Heinemann, who also owned the centre. He had two wives. One fairly young and German with two children, and another who was a bit older, lived in London working as a teacher. She was Pakistani I think and couldn't have children. David invited me to many of the workshops that were held at 'The Rainbow Centre' for free. Workshops on massage, self development and one on the way posture affects your sense of well being. As I got to know David H. he predicted that I was going to be his third wife. I didn't find him attractive. He was short, born a Jew with beard and moustache and was about 40 plus years old, but because of our mutual interest in spirituality we had a good rapport, and conversation flowed liberally between us. David H. also said he was psychic and predicted that I would travel to exotic places and that I would also do a PhD.

I was looking in a window to a book shop by the poly toward the end of term and met a final year student, a black girl called Betty. She seemed a bit frantic at the time and was giving me advice on my years to come at Plymouth. She said something like, "work hard, but don't be too clever. They don't like it when you're too clever. As for me I'm going to Oxford to get married." I can't remember whether she said her husband to be was black or white, and then she said goodbye and was gone. I thought, "How strange. What is she talking about?"

The exams although anxiety inducing, came and went relatively successfully. That is, I passed all of them. Richard hired a van and offered to take Faith and myself home. His friends came to Plymouth to see him off. His friend Antonio was astoundingly good looking. He was mixed race, and although he was very streetwise I was surprised to discover he was a solicitor. He had a baby daughter too but had split up with his baby's mother. Richard said he wasn't going to come back to finish his degree saying he couldn't take much more of Plymouth. We had fun on the journey going back home. They asked me to play my guitar for them to which I consented, and when I played and sang, they all laughed at me. I don't think it was *what* I played, but more the *way* I played and sang that caused the laughter. My singing voice was a far cry from the black female divas that we were all accustomed to hearing, and my guitar strumming was worse than basic. When we got to my parents flat it was late and I nervously got out the van first. I overheard Faith say, "I must see the *house*", which made me even more nervous. I don't know what it was about me that caused so much intrigue. Anyway I reluctantly invited them in for tea and coffee after we had unloaded my stuff, and they declined, stifling laughter.

Toward the end of the summer term in Plymouth, I'd asked my dad to send me current copies of the 'Voice' newspaper so that I could apply for jobs for the summer vacation. Luckily I landed a job with the borough of Tower Hamlets as a Senior Sports Leader on a programme they were running for children over the summer vacation. I was working with one other guy called Ralph in a community centre on an estate in Mile End. He was doing a degree in music at the Guildhall School of Music. It was hard work. The children were real tearaways with so much energy but when events were organised for them, they seemed to settle down. Otherwise it was good fun.

Chapter 8: The nervous tic

In my second year, events took a strange turn. Although I never quite felt as though I belonged to Meenaxi & co.'s group, I hung out with them anyway, but in the second year I was completely ostracised by them. It began by them going silent every time I walked into the room where they were talking, and on one occasion I remember Jane mentioning dandruff, and the whole group giggled. Each time they went out, they stopped asking me if I wanted to come, and pretty soon I had become a social isolate. And it was really significant, because by this time, everyone had formed their cliques on the psychology course and I suppose everyone assumed that my clique was with Meenaxi & co. But when they realized I wasn't hanging out with them, nobody else invited me to join their clique. It was awful.

On more than one occasion I asked Meenaxi what the problem was when we were in of an evening alone. She said nothing was wrong, except on one occasion when she gave an extremely weird answer saying something like, "There are all sorts of reasons why people don't like someone," the rest of her answer being strangely enigmatic. If she was telling me it was because they were envious of me, I found it really difficult to believe. I didn't think I'd given them any reason to be envious of me at all. After all I was the only one in my family that went on to polytechnic, we were extremely poor and they were the ones with the fine straight hair, not me. Anyway, the atmosphere in the flat became really tense. I'd often hear

Meenaxi et al in Meenaxi's room talking and laughing together and it made me feel so lonely. Not only that, going to and from lectures alone was stressful. I felt as though everyone including the lecturers were talking about me because I no longer had a group of friends to hang out with. I went to the student services department for counselling and had a session with a male counsellor. I cried to him, saying no one seemed to like me and I didn't know why. He was sympathetic but at the same time he looked me up and down in what I thought was a sexual way, and made me feel really disconcerted. Sex, or being appealing sexually, was the last thing on my mind in the counselling room at that time. So when I left, I decided I wouldn't go back for any further sessions.

I started looking for alternative accommodation toward Christmas. That really put me out. After all, *I* found the flat at Restormel Terrace first, and I didn't see why I had to leave. But Meenaxi was as stoic as ever bearing the tension and thriving it seemed. I became more and more debilitated and wan as time went by. So much for spirituality. I was suppose to be able to rise above it all, at least accept the situation as the inevitable process of 'involution' that entailed crushing my ego, as it was only when this occurred that you could reach a state called 'mind', 'consciousness' or 'God'. However I couldn't accept it, and I concluded that you couldn't give something up (or crush something), that you didn't have. I decided I didn't have an ego to crush in the first place. So I more or less abandoned my beliefs about spirituality or transcendental psychology.

The psychology course was structured so that you could have a sabbatical year between your second and third year making the course four years in duration. The polytechnic had links with Universities in America, and there was the opportunity to go to America if you chose. I was interested and spoke to my tutor Dave Rose about it at the beginning of my second year. He said it was possible and encouraged me to speak to Maria who was a final year student who had spent a year in America. Maria was a Polish blonde haired girl who was a lesbian. I asked her how her year was in America, and she said it was wonderful, and little else. I felt as though she was lying. She was shaky, and for someone that was suppose to have had a great time, she didn't have much to say. Given the way things were currently going for me and what Maria didn't say about America, I felt as though going abroad would have been a bad idea and didn't give America a second thought.

I attended the African-Caribbean society on one occasion more. A Greek or Turkish girl had been elected in as chair, and it was no longer full of the black faces that I remembered from my first year. There were white people in it. A few months later Nathan, an Asian guy had been elected in as chair. I wondered what had happened. Back at my mums place I discovered she was being overwhelmed by calls for me from Richard's friends. I'm not sure which ones exactly.

I moved house in the spring term of my second year, January '90. It was a street away from Restormel Terrace. The house wasn't as nice as the one at Restormel Terrace and there were more rooms and therefore more students. I thought a great opportunity to make new friends. Anyway

110

when I was moving my stuff in, I was pleasantly surprised to find that Matthew DaRosa was occupying the next room. Great, I thought. A boyfriend perhaps? Nathan was also living in the same house and was good friends with Matthew. The house was freezing. My feet and hands were permanently like blocks of ice. There was no central heating, and my room was attached to a sort of conservatory which I kept my clothes in. This made my bedroom even more cold. There was one other girl in the house and she was dating one of the boys that occupied a room upstairs. There were six of us in the house all together all white British except Nathan and myself. I was vulnerable. I desperately wanted to make new friends, but there I was a second year student who was more or less friendless. I felt this was bound to raise questions with any potential friends. For example everyone made some friends with people on their courses, but I hadn't. Why not? So the people at the house had more or less formed a clique already, and I wasn't really welcome. Whenever I attempted conversation with them, they talked quickly and made no indication that there was a mutual interest. I became paranoid and pressured myself to find things to say to them when I was around them, to avoid an awkward silence. I was usually unsuccessful.

On one occasion I announced to the other students in the house that I was going to have some friends over. I felt, if they saw that I had some friends, I would be more appealing to them and they wouldn't find it so difficult to accept me. I invited none other than Nisha and Meenaxi around who had already made it clear that I was no friend of theirs. But, I was desperate. The same evening that I invited them around, the other girl in the house invited a whole heap of girls from her course over and they laughed and chatted to each other as if we weren't there non stop, the whole evening. I was mortified.

I continued attending and sitting in lectures alone, and in the evening I would skulk into Matthews room and try chatting him up. He showed no signs of succumbing to my overtures, although I did feel he liked me. I became so frustrated at one point that I asked Nathan if Matthew was gay. Anyway, one evening he invited me into his room for a glass of Southern Comfort, and while we listened to music, he lying in his bed mumbled, "Why don't you just come in bed and join me." I asked him to repeat what he said. As desperate as I was, I didn't intend to be anybody's one night stand that they felt embarrassed about the next morning. As it happened he didn't repeat what he said, and that was probably as close to going out with Matthew as I was ever going to get. Occasionally I went out with the people at the house, after all, although it wasn't quite the swinging 60's I was still a student and suppose to be having the time of my life. It wasn't pleasant. Often I'd get left behind, and end up alone, and the bond that the others had between them simply didn't extend to me.

Pretty soon I developed a nervous tic in my eye. Whenever I spoke to someone, I felt my eye twitching away and that I imagined gave everything away about the desperation of my situation. I became paranoid and developed a mild stammer. I also started suffering from insomnia and constipation. I couldn't believe what was happening to me. My dandruff didn't go away either, and whenever people were standing behind me, I felt as though they could see how bad my dandruff was. This was particularly true in lectures where the seats were tiered. Not long after people actually started doing things behind my back, wherever I went around the poly. I remember on one occasion, students from the psychology course had arranged to meet at the Union and were then to go onto one of the night clubs in Plymouth. I had been invited. I was really excited, because I thought this would give me the opportunity to mingle with the other students in an informal setting and possibly join in on one of their cliques. Anyway somehow I wound up on the dance floor of the Warehouse nightclub with Nisha and Meenaxi. There I was dancing away when we were joined by two white girls who Nisha seemed to know. They were standing behind me, and as I was dancing, they started doing something behind my back. I could tell because the people in front of me just smiled emptily at me occasionally looking at the girls behind me. When I turned around to see what was going on, they started laughing at one another and carried on dancing like two schoolgirls who had been caught doing something naughty. Like a shadow, the humiliation of what had just occurred swept over me. I imagined everyone in the nightclub who wasn't dancing or who was dancing nearby, had seen what had taken place and the thought of this simply added weight to the shame that I felt. I had done nothing wrong, yet it was me that carried the shame, not the two white girls. It went on. The bad intended carry on behind my back I mean. Every time someone did something behind me it was like my head was pulled back as if there were something connecting the back of my head to them, and once this had occurred, my heart sank, a deep depression settling over me. I stopped going to the Union to avoid the torment that went alongside someone doing something behind my back.

On another occasion at the Rizzy nightclub, I bumped into Steve Russ. We danced the night away together. We even danced to the slow record at the end when most of the students cleared the dance floor. At this point Andy, Steve's friend from the psychology course, came up to Steve and said, "You're mad." Steve asked me what he meant by saying that, to which I told him I didn't know. That night Steve came back to our house with me. I thought the competition might push Matthew into action. Steve was uncomfortable when he saw Matthew, but he spent half the night in my room anyway, and half way through the night got up to go back to his place. We didn't have sex.

Things came to a bit of a head when I was living in that house. One day I was in my room attempting to do some work with my bedroom door open. The living room door was open too so that I could hear the TV. I liked it that way. It made me feel comfortable and relaxed and not so isolated. Anyway there were two people in the living room, and one of them shut the living room door. I went and opened it again and then went back to my room. A little while later, they shut the door again. It was awful because I felt as though they were shutting the door to shut me out. I went and opened the door again and went back to my room and broke down crying wondering what I was going to do. I ran out of the house to the nearest phone box and called Janet. Although I wasn't close to her, I'd kept in touch with her from the African-Caribbean society. I burbled to Janet down the phone, "I've got to get out of this house. I'm not getting on with the other students." She came over immediately and said there was a spare room in her house and that I could move in with them. So I did.

Janet's house was in Ladysmith Avenue about 15 to 20 minutes from the poly. It was centrally heated and like me Janet felt the cold bitterly in winter and as she and Saheed took charge of the house, the heating was always turned up, so it was always warm. Saheed was Indian and also Janet's boyfriend. They had neighbouring rooms downstairs. My room was upstairs along with the other students who lived in the house. There was a patio at the back of the house too which meant we could have barbecues and lie out there in the summer. Apart from my housing situation which afforded me a little more comfort, nothing improved for me. I became nervous and shaky in addition to having a stammer and a nervous tic. It was Janet that pointed out one day that I was ruining my complexion. I started getting pimples on my forehead which simply wouldn't go away. So I picked them, and they left little black marks. I remember in a computing session one day, there were a couple of us to a computer and it was my turn to do the exercise that we had been assigned. I had combed my hair into two cane rows, so that there was a parting down the middle. The two lecturers that were giving the session came up behind me and looked in my hair. I turned around to catch them grimacing at each other. Once again humiliation swept over me. People on my course who I had formed fleeting acquaintances with pretended nothing was happening. I asked George (a girl) if my nervous tic was bad one day, and she said, "No it isn't", as though I were imagining the whole thing. One morning I was scheduled for a social psychology lecture. I went into the lecture theatre and sat right next to a girl I hardly ever spoke to. I'm not sure what possessed me to do it. I just suddenly thought maybe it *was* my imagination that I was being excluded by everyone, and if I acted as though nothing were wrong maybe I'd be ok. Anyway this girl shrunk away from me which made me even more nervous and made my eye twitch more ferociously. To compound the matter, during the lecture which was given by Fraser Reid, he mentioned all in the context of the lecture he was giving, that if 'they' don't like you, you should leave. I was sure he was talking about me, and this wasn't the first lecture that made me feel this way. There were innuendos in practically every lecture I attended, but this one pushed me, already in a fragile state, over the edge. I left the lecture before it ended and tears streaming down my face, ran home.

When I got home, Janet was in her room getting ready to go to a lecture. I threw myself on the floor in her room and screamed, "I can't take any more! Just take me to hospital." I was crying frantically. Janet, who was the course rep. in the second year of her biology degree spoke to me matter of factly. She said, "You just need some counselling Rosie, then you'll be alright." So the following day I went to the student services department and asked to see a *female* counsellor. I had counselling sessions every week, and in addition I stopped attending lectures. I didn't give a thought to the work I'd be missing and the exams at the end of the year. Attending lectures and being around the polytechnic had become a major stressor for me. I simply couldn't face it. I spent most of my time in bed reflecting on what had taken place over the past year. If nothing else, this seemed to ease the nervous tic in my eye which was particularly bad when I attempted to interact with others. I really couldn't comprehend why this was happening to me. I felt as though I was a likable person, and I hadn't done anything wrong to upset anybody, yet, here I was being ostracized. It hurt like mad. Whenever I was in a public place I became paranoid about people standing behind me and had a panic attack.

I found out that Man Yee and Gemma had joined the Duke of Edinburgh Award Scheme. They said it was really good and that I should join. This wasn't an invitation to friendship. They kept their distance. Anyway I joined the scheme, and on a couple of occasions we went camping on Dartmoor. Once during a thunder storm. It was lambing season and I gather the lambs had come early as they were littered across the moor dead, without a parent nearby. It was a traumatic sight. It wasn't the first time I'd been to Dartmoor since being in Plymouth. In the first year occasionally I went for walks there with a couple of mature students Mike McKay being one of them. He used to work on the stock market, made lots of money, travelled a great deal, and then I gather things went wrong for him. He left his job and decided to do a degree. He was white working class, but not from London. I remember we walked into the firing range of the army once, completely oblivious to this fact. A soldier came up to us on horse back and enlightened us.

Over the Easter vacation, I went home for about a week. I didn't stay any longer than that because my mum had a relative staying in my room from St. Lucia which meant I had to sleep in the living room. I couldn't handle that at that time. I was extremely sensitized to the world and I needed my privacy, so shortly after I went back to

Plymouth. I discovered Janet had come back early too. She had similar problems to me at her mothers place. Her mother had let her room to a French girl. She was as angry as I was about my mum. Anyway, we had a heart to heart about our respective families and I learned that she used to get beaten quite severely by her father. One morning, I went to the toilet as I usually did and then like a bolt out of the blue I was paralysed by paroxysms of pain through my bowel. Each wave of pain forced me to grip myself and stop me in my tracks. It was the same pain I experienced before I left Stratford, London, to come to Plymouth only it went on for much longer. I was screaming and crying in tormented agony. Janet accompanied me to my doctor where I was subjected to an anal examination. I was frightened. I thought there was something severely wrong with me. The doctor said he couldn't find any obstructions in my bowel and that there didn't appear to be anything wrong. He simply suggested I eat lots of high fibre foods, and sent me away. The pains lasted for the whole day, waning as the day wore on.

Like a magnet, in spite of the fact that I was more or less a social outcast, I was still drawn by the nightclubs, hanging on to the hope that my fate might change somehow. So almost weekly, along with Janet and Adam (one of the other residents in the house), we went to the Rizzy nightclub. It was usually when we were around others in public places that I experienced Janet's disregard. She would talk incessantly to whoever we were with as if I wasn't there or we would be dancing together on the dance floor when she would suddenly without any warning, walk off leaving me dancing by myself. Maybe it was because I was insecure that this upset me, but for me the fun of going

out to a nightclub was that it was a shared experience
between like minded friends. She was a fantastic dancer
though. And that was another thing, whenever I asked her
to teach me some of her moves she always shrugged me off
saying that it was easy. It was incidents like this that
continually pushed me to the edge. I was chatted up by a
guy at the Rizzy nightclub one night. He offered to buy me
a drink, and then we arranged to meet each other in the city
centre the following day. Whether I found him attractive
or not, didn't come into it. I thought I was onto a winner.
Janet was always telling me if I had a boyfriend I wouldn't
have half the problems I was experiencing. Half way
through my drink, John a student I had met after being left
stranded when out with my previous house share one night,
came up to me and whispered, "Are you mad? He's a
squaddie," and walked away. I wondered how he could
tell, not that it made any difference to me. I was warned
about the sailors in Plymouth before I came to the poly,
and I envisaged a lot of young men in the traditional navy
blue and white uniform by the sea front. But the armed
forces were much less visible than I had expected.

Faith came to see Janet at our house one day. She barely
acknowledged me, referring to me while talking to Janet
with a giggle as 'that coconut'. I was incensed and
expressed my indignation to Faith, but the label echoed in
my head. I thought that's why this is happening to me,
because I'm not like Janet or Faith or other black girls, I'm
different. Gabriela came to see me from London while I
was sharing that house with Janet and co. We went to a
club together while she was with us and Janet's comment
about Gabriela was, "You're safe," the intimation being
that I wasn't. I recalled Janet telling me about something

that happened to her in a lecture once. She said this guy made a slight against her, or something like that, in front of everyone. Anyway she harboured her anger until the lecture was over and then when she got the opportunity, she warned him and told him never to do that to her again. She *threatened* him. When she told me, I looked on at her with admiration. I thought, that's what I needed to do to anyone that did something to me behind my back, but I just couldn't bring myself to react. I thought it would backfire.

I realized around exam time toward the end of the summer term that I was going to have problems with the exams as I had missed so many of the lectures, and had no notes to revise from. I invited Man Yee and her partner around for dinner and asked her if I could copy her notes. Without the slightest objection, she consented, and that made me feel a whole lot more settled. I copied the computing assignment from Andy, Steve's friend, along with practically everyone else on the course. All the psychology students seemed to have problems with computing. However when the exams were over, *I* and only I was accused of plagiarism by the lecturer Paul Kenyon who was in charge of the computing assignment. I complained to my tutor explaining that I was hardly the only one that copied the assignment. But he insisted that it was only me. Saheed, Janet and a friend of theirs from the island of St. Vincent said that it was racism and that I should write to the Commission for Racial Equality. However, I didn't. Janet would often say to me that my problem was that I was colour blind and that I had better be careful otherwise I would end up bitter and twisted. I was set another assignment that I had to complete by January '91, but apart from that I scraped through all of the exams. However given that the second year exam results and coursework assignments went toward your final degree result, my performance which was about average meant that I had to kiss goodbye to any hopes of mine for an upper second or first class degree. This meant that my aspiration to become a Clinical Psychologist just like the majority of students on the course, had more or less been quashed.

I kept in touch with Maria, the final year student who said she had a good time in America. Like me, she was having quite a rough time socially, however she seemed to retaliate against her fate where as I was locked in an endless cycle of wondering why this was happening to me, and analysing my past and my behaviour to see whether there were any clues. In response to being ostracized by the students on her course, Maria decided *she didn't like* the students. Her social milieu consisted of a few social drop outs i.e. punks who lived in squats and didn't work and some lesbian women who she'd met around Plymouth. She also attended a spiritual church which was full of mediums. She said they told her she was going to be rich and they gave her a message from her grandmother who had passed away. Her situation had reached a boiling point around the time of her final year exams. Apparently she spoke to her friends about ending her life often and she had issues with her Catholic upbringing and her father. Her friends informed the social services department, and she was sectioned in a psychiatric hospital.

Once again before I had left Plymouth to go back to London, I'd asked my father to send me copies of the Voice Newspaper so that I could apply for jobs over the summer. I came across an advertisement for a college in

Birmingham that held residential courses for mature students over a period of one year for people wanting to study the humanities. The courses were being held at Fircroft College which was based at the Cadbury's House in Birmingham and was affiliated in some way to Birmingham University. I thought this was exactly what I needed. I felt I lacked an understanding of the processes which occur in society and the language used to explain these processes. I felt this course would put all my wrongs right. I wouldn't have to pay anything for the course either, as there was a body that awarded bursaries to anyone that was accepted on the course. I was invited to the Cadbury's House for an interview. It was beautiful. There were tennis courts in the grounds, and on arrival I saw two white girls decked in long flowing skirts, shawls and hair flowing, wondering through the grounds with tennis rackets. The house itself was surrounded by fields, and was built in Tudor style and it was tremendously peaceful. I was given a room for the night in preparation for my interview in the morning, so I took the liberty of wondering through the house that evening. It was breathtaking, and there was a piano in the dining room which I imagined of an evening we could congregate around and sing songs. I was completely taken by the scene and I thought I was bound to heal here. I was interviewed by several lecturers who, given that I was already at polytechnic and therefore not the typical candidate for the Cadbury's House, were very nice. I stumbled and stuttered with my words trying to explain why the course would be valuable for me. I was well received. I was offered a place, but it was dependent on my obtaining an academic reference for the bursary. I gave my tutor Dave Rose as my referee and I don't know what he said to them, but they wouldn't award me a bursary. And so I didn't go to the Cadbury's House in Birmingham.

I was unsuccessful at finding a job in the Voice Newspaper, but I decided that I needed to get back to my roots and be around local people, the people of Hackney, London. So I applied to none other than Sainsbury's supermarket for a job. I decided there was no way I could survive another year at poly so I thought I'd take a year out to see if my fate might change. It wasn't going to be a very constructive year out. Most students, if they were taking a year out got placements in the field they intended to work in when they graduated. My circumstances hadn't afforded me the privilege of that degree of organisation. My year out was simply going to be some breathing space for me.

Chapter 9: Ice

Guedelia, my relative who was staying with my mum from St. Lucia had moved on into her own flat. It meant that I had my room back at my mum's place which I was grateful for. I started working at Sainsbury's in July '90. I wasn't the only student to be working there, there were a few of us. We were given a health questionnaire to fill in with the application form, and on it I indicated that I suffered from nervousness. Later I realized that that was a really stupid thing to have done because the personnel department wrote to my doctor asking them to clarify the matter. Anyway it turns out that my doctor, Sam Heard, told my sister who was working at the surgery that I had an abortion, and that I said to my employer that I suffered from nervousness. Well apparently I learned that you don't say things like that on health questionnaires unless they are confirmed medical conditions. But the truth is, I really did feel that my nervousness was becoming a medical condition, although I didn't say anything to anyone. My mum found out about the abortion too. I quelled any questions by kicking up a fuss about the fact that Dr Heard had no right discussing my medical records with anyone other than myself, and that was that. Other than that working at Sainsbury's was alright. I made friends with an African Christian girl there called Bola. We ate at each others place when my mum had gone on holiday to St. Lucia with Claudia. She invited me to her church, telling me that I was missing out as Jesus was a great saviour. I went along to her church with her one Sunday and at the end of the service she prayed over me the prayer of salvation and when she'd finished she looked at me ecstatically saying, "You've been saved, you've been saved! How do you feel?" Well I gather I was suppose to have been transformed by the presence of Christ in me as Bola had been and most of the people at her church, but I felt no change whatsoever. My cylinders were still burning low. There were a few other Africans who I shared my lunch hours and breaks with at Sainsbury's. They made my time there all the more pleasant, as I was more or less ostracized by the rest of the staff. I put this down to the fact that the referee I gave to Sainsbury's i.e. my tutor Dave Rose, must have given a poor reference and spoken to them about my experience in Plymouth. I couldn't think of any other reason.

Alex, another cousin who had recently come from St. Lucia was dating a Ghanaian girl Sophie Amedume. She was really nice, and we became quite good friends. We went out clubbing together, and she introduced me to her friends and cousins at a cultural / fashion show. Apart from Sophie, I continued to see Cheryl and occasionally I went out with my nieces Jessica and Gabriela. I joined a black women's self awareness group that was being held in a women's centre in Hampstead not long after I arrived back from Plymouth and in addition I bought many self help psychology books and continued analysing myself and trying to discover why living was going so badly wrong for me.

I was determined to make a go of things so I tried extending my social circle through work. Alongside my job at Sainsbury's I got a series of part time jobs one after the other that entailed working evenings and weekends. Each ended miserably. First was a job as a bar maid in a trendy pub not far from Sainsbury's near Dalston Junction called the Trolley Stop. I went there on one occasion with Tania and a few of her friends, decided I liked it thinking it would be a good place to make friends, and applied for a job there. I was accepted right away without references. For my first few evenings there, things went along swimmingly. I got on with the other bartenders ok, and I was well received by the punters. However I think it was on my fourth night there, events took a strange turn. It was a Saturday night I believe and the pub was packed. The other bartenders both men and women ganged up on me literally. The pub owners happened to be away on this occasion. Every time I turned my back to the other bartenders, they did monkey movements behind me, and implied I smelled every time I lifted my arm to draught a drink for a customer by wafting their nose. Panic struck. I don't know how I survived the evening without screaming or having a nervous breakdown, but I did. At one point I excused myself to make a phone call. I wanted to see if I could get one of my brothers or sisters to witness the carry on behind the bar so that if I pulled them up about it, I'd have someone to back me up. However everyone I called was out or busy, and too preoccupied to notice the distress in my voice. The punters simply looked on without breathing a word. I busied myself collecting glasses and emptying ash trays in an attempt to prove to everyone that I did not smell. The whole evening was a nightmare. I didn't go back to work at that pub, but the following day I went to see the pub owners and indicated that something was amiss the previous night, without giving any detail. They weren't very sympathetic and I got the feeling they were aware of what had taken place.

I had two other part time jobs after working at the Trolley Stop, both lasting only a few weeks. First was a job as a waitress at a new black owned and run jazz bar/restaurant in Dalston Lane called Pamela's. The minute I found out about it I thought I had to get a job there as I only lived down the road and thought I was bound to make some really nice friends while at the same time mingling with other black people. Ian was the owner, and Pamela who the place was named after was the head waitress. For the short time that I was there, Pamela made my life hell. She was constantly at my throat telling me how the job should be done. It all climaxed when I went there to work one evening and the three other waitresses including Pamela and a new white girl they'd employed, stood in front of me with foundation plastered on their faces like they were trying to make a point. For whatever reason, my life was distressing and I guess that took its toll on my complexion. My clear spotless complexion of my first year and prior to my first year in Plymouth had given way to pimples that I picked at causing then to leave black marks, and I had shadows around my mouth and beneath my eyes. If Pamela was trying to tell me something about my complexion, why didn't she attempt to have a girly chat with me? Anyway, after that I felt completely excluded. After all, I was a black girl, why was she, another black woman treating me like this? I left shortly after, and on walking past the restaurant on one occasion saw a black woman working there who didn't have foundation packed on her face. I wondered about Pamela.

At about this time, at the Fridge nightclub in Brixton with Cheryl one evening, we met a couple of students. White boys middle class, out to have a good time, as we were.

They both made a bee line for me, the quieter blonde one having got to me first, pushed the more extrovert one off. I preferred the looks of the latter, but didn't have the eloquence to wheedle my way into his presence and thought anyway, seeing as I couldn't speak without stuttering, I was probably better off with the quiet one who was called James. I spoke little and at every opportunity danced the night away hoping that my dancing would make up for my dim wit. At the end of the night he invited me to a party in Chelsea the following week, telling me he would pick me up at a nearby station. I agreed, so met him at the appointed time at the station, the following week. Apart from the fact that I didn't speak much, the party was going well until the conversation somehow switched on to aromatherapy oils which I had used before. I said something about aromatherapy oils being great except that they had no effect. I was living evidence of this. Who was I to speak? Both James and a blonde girl jumped down my throat insisting that aromatherapy oils were potent medicinal oils. I stuck to my guns albeit weakly while the other too more or less said I was stupid. The party soured. Then as though to make amends, the blonde girl said to me that she was only going out with her boyfriend because his father was a famous artist. I forget which, and then she made a joke about James's name. He was called James Joyce. I nodded as though I knew what she was talking about, but they both knew I didn't. James exasperated shouted at me, "You know, the author?" I didn't. Nerves wreaked havoc with my stomach again and I fell silent, everyone else babbling on as though I wasn't there. My fate had been decided. I looked down at what I was wearing. At the beginning of the night I thought I looked pretty cool wearing black leggings, a short dress that flared out at the hips made from fabric that was printed with a new age image of the sun, a pair of black socks that I wore gathered around my ankles, and monkey boots. Now I felt dishevelled, and all I saw was the specs of fluff on my socks and I wondered why I hadn't noticed it at the beginning of the night. I felt awful. After a little while I told James I wanted to go home. He got us a cab, and all the way back to my mother's place, we were silent. I barely said goodbye when I got out of the mini cab. He seemingly with a disgusted countenance, muttered something at me and closed the cab door and that was the last I saw of James.

While still working at Sainsbury's daytime, my second part time job was at Sadler's Wells Theatre at weekends working at the stand during intervals that sold programmes and theatre paraphernalia. Once again, for some reason I didn't gel with the other theatre assistants. They were chatty and happy and I felt like a dark cloud in their presence. There was one other black girl who was doing a degree in music. I thought that we could become friends seeing as we shared ethnic origin and were both doing degrees, although not in the same subject. But I had no such luck. She simply didn't warm to me, like everyone else. The stand that I worked in was organised so that the paraphernalia I sold was displayed on a wall behind me. One evening during an interval while I was working, two blonde girls came up to the stand and just stood close by. Whenever somebody asked me the price of an ornament or piece of jewellery which entailed me having to turn my back to them, the two blonde girls started to carry on behind my back. Once again like a fox trapped in a snare, the anxiety rose in me as I thought wildly about what I

could do, surrounded by all of these people. I tried to catch
the attention of one of the other theatre assistants, but she
was busy seeing to peoples coats in the cloakroom.
Surrounded by all of these people, I was completely and
totally without an ally who could look out for me. At the
end of the evening, at the top of the stairs leading to the
foyer, dressed in a slinky sky blue dress, I saw a blonde
girl that was at the Laban Centre when I was there. She
was brilliant at the Laban Centre, and she looked good that
evening at Sadler's Wells. I couldn't help but think about
how different our lives were. I didn't go back to work at
the theatre after that night. I thought another evening like
that would really push me over the edge, into madness.
Nervous and living in somewhat unstable and strange
conditions, I clung on to my sanity.

The black women's group ran once a week for about 12
weeks. I actually felt quite comfortable there. None of the
women seemed like typical black women i.e. loud and
aggressive and a few even had what I felt were 'coconut'
qualities. Even so they didn't warm to me like I expected
them to. I was as unreserved as I could be yet they all
seemed to keep their distance bar one. October Tempest.
She was Nigerian, and wore a very poorly attached weave
that revealed her natural hair, and fell down past her
shoulders. When I got to know her, she said she wore her
hair long because people respond differently to you if you
have long hair. She was very articulate, and exuded
confidence, nevertheless she often referred to her male
English guardian who took her into shops she felt
intimidated by, even though she must have been in her
thirties at least. Sex for her was simply something that
satisfied a physical need. Talibah the course facilitator

agreed with her! As we both lived in Hackney, we got the train home together. It was then that I decided she must be a prostitute. She sat with her legs open, and was totally uninhibited. Ok, so she was wearing a pair of leggings, but she just seemed past caring. We went out a couple of times together anyway. For a meal at a Thai restaurant in Stoke Newington where she was known by the waitresses, and a couple of times to the Fridge night club in Brixton where just like Janet, she deserted me to explore the social arena. She invited me to a wedding of a friend or relative of hers too and would you believe we were given a lift by the chauffeur in the wedding couples Rolls Royce to the Fridge night club, him saying he had Diana Ross in the back seat! Anyway I decided my notions about her being a prostitute were confirmed when she called me one Saturday to ask me if I wanted to meet a male friend of hers at a party she was having. She said he was white, very good looking, and she thought we'd get on really well. I declined the offer. That wasn't all. I went to her flat once and I think she'd been crying. She looked really distraught and harped on about life being so awful. For some reason I felt as though she'd been slapped around by someone. I decided her pimp. Her flat was chic. At least the front room was anyway, but her bedroom was dark, dingy and untidy. The friendship didn't last. The last I heard of her was when I answered an ad placed in the Voice newspaper from a facilitator of a therapy group. She was the person on the other end of the phone, and although we didn't overtly acknowledge each other, we both knew who we were talking to.

I often wondered how circumstances had followed me from Plymouth to London. I concluded at Plymouth on the polytechnic campus that rumours had been spread about me having dandruff, and this is what caused people to carry on behind my back. It started with people looking into my hair behind me I guess to check if the rumours were true, and progressed on to them more or less acting like fools behind me, although while it happened, I couldn't rationalize it like this. Instead I became more and more wound up and humiliated by it. However London was a much bigger place and relations between people are not as intimate as they were at the polytechnic, so I wondered why people were carrying on whenever I had my back turned to them. I thought, having dabbled in spirituality that it had something to do with my aura. I felt spiritually that I was willing these experiences upon myself perhaps. However, I finally decided that the source was my references from the polytechnic to prospective employers. Somehow my referees conveyed my experiences at the polytechnic to them and my current employers took it upon themselves to carry on in the same vein. At the time, I could think of no other explanation.

Like my skin, I felt the stress that I was under had also taken its toll on my hair. My hair became brittle, wiry and broke more than usual. In addition although I know afro hair is frizzy, it was even more frizzy now. My sister Francesca suggested I get it relaxed. She had her hair relaxed. Prior to this I'd heard from so many black girls that relaxing your hair ruins it, and that it was definitely not something that I should do particularly, they said, as I had such beautiful hair already. I'd think to myself, yeah, right! Anyway, I went along with my sister's suggestion, and one day she came over with one box of a Dark and Lovely relaxor kit and proceeded to relax my hair. Half way through, she ran out of relaxor, and only half of my hair was done, so she went to Ridley Road market to get another box, while I waited in, my scalp burning away. I was astounded by the results when she'd finished. For the first time in my life I could feel the shape of my scalp through my hair and my hair actually *hung* down straight to my shoulders. I felt beautiful even though that wasn't what the world was telling me, and I thought, so this is how white girls feel. The burning of my scalp revealed itself in the following days. Huge scabs had formed on my scalp and clumped my hair together in places. Even so, it didn't stop me enjoying the feeling of my hair being blown about by the wind. My hair didn't stop breaking, and my dandruff didn't magically disappear either as I thought it would for some reason. The scabs came away from my scalp, making it look as though I was suffering from a severe case of psoriasis. I became even more self conscious about people standing behind me. But when the scabs cleared away I thought I looked ok. I plastered my hair with grease whenever I washed it thinking this would stop it from breaking.

Although I lived approximately 15 minutes away from Sainsbury's on foot, that didn't stop me arriving late most days. Often I hitched lifts on Queensbridge Road to work. Mr Oxley was the store manager, and I felt he had a soft spot for me. When a vacancy arose in the cash office, he offered it to me. Pleasant as it was being away from the shop floor, it meant I came under the autocratic glare of Anne, a white woman in her fifties. She made working in the cash office really uncomfortable, and at least once I caught her grimacing at the scabs resembling large flakes of dandruff in my hair. I mean, it wasn't like I was the only black girl there. This was Dalston for goodness's sakes! But for various reasons unclear to me I was a social stigma. This didn't stop me flirting with men, typically white, who I found attractive even though I could barely speak without stammering or getting unrealistically nervous. There was this guy that I really liked called Tony. He reminded me of a student that I was infatuated about back in Plymouth called Glyn who was a sort of 'Jesus Jones' character. I didn't even get to know Glyn, but with Tony, I decided I wouldn't let a good opportunity pass me by. We'd arranged to go out for a drink one evening, to the Trolley Stop (before I started working there as a bar maid), and that day I bumped into Tony coming back from lunch. He was carrying a small packet in a paper bag given by a chemist. I was convinced they were condoms, and I thought to myself, I barely know this guy and he has sex in mind already! Besides, he'd already told me that he had a girlfriend. However that didn't stop me snogging him at the station while we were waiting for his train to come on the way home. In the process a gang of black youths passed us by and snatched my bag exclaiming, "You can't do that in Hackney!" They took my purse but I managed to recover my bag which was dumped further on down the street. Tony's comment to me was, "That's bad man. On your own turf!"

I got my nose pierced in the winter of '90, something I'd been dwelling on for some time. Although I wasn't overtly a Madonna fan, I thought she was pretty good at what she did and initially I guess it was her influence that encouraged the nose piercing. Whenever I could, I went out clubbing with Cheryl mostly who had by now graduated with a 2:2, but occasionally my niece Jessica who was about two years my junior. Usually the evening was marred by someone doing something behind my back which set my thoughts off onto the interminable questioning of *why*? I still hadn't really told anyone about it. I attempted to tell Dorothy my niece at a family party my mum gave after the Sadlers Wells job, but she just laughed it away as if it were nothing saying, "They're only doing it to you because you're on your own." I wasn't consoled. You see as far as my family were concerned I was their pride and joy. At least my parents'. I was at university. Well not quite. When they spoke to me or of me, they were filled with promise. Even though it was pretty obvious that things were not going as they should have been, and I was not as happy as I should have been, I couldn't bring myself to explain the madness that I was going through. I mean, who were all these strangers who I'd never seen in my life who seemingly had a slight against me? I couldn't work it out, and there was no way that anyone in my family were going to either. Each had problems of their own and particularly with my sisters, these problems usually entailed their partners.

Clinton, my sister Justine's partner, and the father of her last two children Delroy and Natalie, had a nervous breakdown. Justine had moved to a council house in Dalston Junction by this time. Apparently she told him she didn't want him anymore and he simply retreated into himself, started talking to himself and babbled on about nothing that made sense every time you tried to have a conversation with him. He spent most of the rest of his life sitting near Dalston Junction station strumming on a guitar. Whenever anyone in the family came across him they talked about how embarrassing it was as he always tried to talk to them. My heart broke when I first heard about him. I was convinced if I had gotten to him sooner, before the insanity became entrenched, he wouldn't be mad. Francesca bought a house with her partner at about this time too, but it got repossessed because her partner walked out on her and she couldn't afford to pay the mortgage. When Claudia went to St. Lucia with her children and my mum, I bumped into Taylor (Claudia's husband) a couple of times. Things weren't going well for him at work. In him I saw the same panic that I felt at losing control of circumstances, of having the unexpected happen. He was working for Cable TV and for some reason or other the manager (an American) was breathing down his neck. He said there was another black woman who worked there who he thought would empathise with him, but it seemed *she* was doing just fine and she wasn't concerned about anyone else. Anyway he invited me to an evening out with his work mates that I guess he felt obliged to attend. We went to the Theatre but I don't recall what we saw. I was too taken aback by Taylor's manager who was a fat American and although I only spoke to him for a short while, noted his acridity. The whole evening made me very nervous. Taylor was all fingers and thumbs and smiles. When we left, he asked me if I could understand what he'd been explaining to me. I told him that he should leave.

Jessica was hanging out with a white girl who I'm pretty sure was a prostitute. Around Christmas time, I cycled over to her place which was then a flat share in Stoke Newington. Wearing bright red lipstick and nail polish I stopped off at a newsagent on Queensbridge Road to buy some sweets. Would you believe Dr Sam Heard walked in.

Flushed with self consciousness and nerves I was reminded of how attractive I found him and became aware only of his intense glare. We exchanged a few words and in no time at all, the moment was gone. Relieved to be out of the shop, I went on my way. That evening, and on a couple of other evenings, Jessica and I roamed the streets of Hackney sometimes dithering outside a nightclub or rave while we decided whether we were going in or not, otherwise chatting men up and searching for some excitement.

Central to my thinking at this time, was what I felt was a lacking in my intellect. There I was, an undergraduate with a mild stammer and a nervous tic in my eye, never mind the constant feeling of anxiety at my centre. It seemed as though everyone that I came into contact with was eloquent, fast talking, and interesting (that is had something to say about everything). I had read a lot of books, and was doing a degree, I felt surely that should give me something to say? Instead however I became obsessed with how quickly and confidently people spoke, and the more I noticed this, the more nervous I became. Whenever I got caught up in an interaction with someone I spent the whole time trying to escape from them, before I stammered or before they noticed how stupid I was. The world seemed to be hurtling by me. I felt like a lamb among wolves. Nobody was gentle or sensitive, everyone was sharp and ruthless. I felt as though I was at everybody's mercy. I was defenceless. It was in this desperate state that during a conversation with Cheryl I took up a suggestion of hers. She said in the worldly manner that was her way, "If I were you, I would sleep with as many men as possible." Up until this point, I still held sex as sacred. That is before I engaged in a sexual relationship I felt there should be some sort of commitment between individuals. I had to feel the relationship was going somewhere. However, on the brink of insanity, my reasoning abandoned me. Like someone that had been hypnotized, I thought it a good idea. My mind was too clouded to even consider whether Cheryl was following her own advice. Come New Years Eve I found myself in a pub, The Kings Head in Stratford with Cheryl, and one of her friends. At midnight we were propositioned by two white men. There was a party in their house which was further up the Romford Road. We lapped up the attention and went along with them. It wasn't much of a party. There were a handful of male and female students about our age. Cheryl gassed on to a couple of the women, I smiled sweetly while talking as little as possible to the more handsome of the two guys that picked us up from the pub who from the start, had made a beeline for me. He lapped it up. He and I escaped to his room not long after, and me barely noticing the sore on his chin, he groped and snogged me, the occasional titter escaping from him. For the lack of a condom, we did not have sex.

The following morning, I felt good, however as the day wore on, there was a niggling sensation on my chin which I scratched. The sensation erupted into a sore. I'd had cold sores before when I was seeing Perry and I was always the first to say to him, "don't kiss me or you'll catch my cold sore." Not that he ever listened. But for some reason, the sore on this guy's chin simply didn't register when I met him. Anyway it seemed I'd caught *something* from him on New Years Day, in the early hours of the morning. As the days progressed, the sore spread in patches from my chin to my cheeks and forehead, and continually itched. It also irritated my eyes. I felt like a diseased animal. The doctor that I saw said it was nothing to worry about, and that it would clear up eventually. When I attempted to get in touch with the culprit again to ask him why he'd been so irresponsible, following some confusion with another of his flatmates who shared the same name, I was always told he was out with his girlfriend.

Apart from sporadically lapsing into meat eating with a ferocity surpassing that of a carnivore, I maintained a healthy vegetarian diet. I decided it was important that I eat well given that I was so stressed. With this in mind, I attended an open evening at the Community Health Foundation then in Old Street where there were samples of macrobiotic cooking and Tai-Chi classes. They had a health food shop and restaurant where I ate occasionally when I was doing O level dance at City and Islington College, Barbican site in 1985. Anyway, at the open evening, as if I were about to steal the crown jewels and was found out, I was met with a contempt unrivalled by that which Hitler would have felt for me. Everyone was hostile. The facilitators eyed me suspiciously, the other participants didn't look at or talk to me at all, and in the Tai-Chi class the woman in front of me attempted to push me out of the way. Ok, so I was the only black person there, but that was no excuse. This was London '91! Through all of this I yearned for Perry. I wondered whether he thought about me as much as I thought about him.

In the new year I landed a new job. It was with a black arts organisation called Pyramid Arts Development and was based in Ashwin Street near to Dalston Junction. The three black women who interviewed me for the job were dressed in bright colours and looked really friendly. I was completely open with them at the interview explaining that I didn't have much experience in this field but I would give it my best shot. Surprisingly, they offered me the post of administrator and truly I thought my troubles would be over. I expected communication to come easily, thought the anxiety would pass and I'd see an end to the carry on behind my back cushioned by like minded black people. Well, I was mistaken. I'd barely gotten through my first day when Judith the manager who also interviewed me, standing behind me in the reception area with Kevin Jones (one of the others in the organisation), came up close behind me and peered into my hair. As usual, as though there were daggers attached to her eyes that stabbed my head when she did this, I felt a tug inside of me and drowning in the familiar feelings of despair that followed, I looked around to see her smiling and chatting to Kevin Jones as though nothing had happened. That wasn't all. At the first staff meeting I attended, whenever I went to say something, Judith interrupted. Everyone else was pretty eloquent. Sensing Judith's hostility and gripped by anxiety, I clammed up. Staff meetings became an event that I dreaded as each time I'd wrack my brains for something innovative to contribute to prove my worth to the others. As far as I can recall, I barely said a word. To be honest, I didn't feel I was that good at the job. My typing skills were poor and at the time I wasn't a great communicator so I couldn't even win favour socially let alone professionally. Kevin Jones was another who made me very nervous. He was a fast talker, like a salesman, and every so often he would suggest something that I should look into now that I was the administrator for the company.

If I felt inadequate in the job, he made me feel ten times worse. He took me along to meet the architects who were responsible for the building refurbishment programme at Pyramid. I was a wreck. I felt as though this whole business was way above my head, and I didn't have a clue. Just introducing myself to them made me stammer and shake visibly.

It was Judith who suggested Victor and I become an item, as we were both unattached. Victor, alongside Kevin Jones, ran the small record label that was attached to Pyramid. He listened to hardcore rap and heavy metal most days, detested white people and had extremely strong views on the way the black community should be led. He once said to me if he had his way he would shoot all the liberals (meaning socialists I believe) in the black community. He said they were responsible for the state of the black community today. So, as I was being paid more than him, we went Dutch on a meal in an African restaurant in Dalston. Thus began my exposure to an African consciousness of sorts. Inwardly I attributed the blame for my negative experiences to white people although I was confused by it all and when black people seemed to participate, felt even more so. I was astounded at how much Victor knew and even more astounded at the fact that he took it for granted that everything that we were exposed to through the media particularly regarding Africa or people of the African Diaspora was a lie. When I asked him how he arrived at his views, he said he reads. Uncannily we had similar past experiences. He was living in some sort of half way house with his family at one stage and ended up having a relationship with a white German woman, much older than him. Through her he came to listen to the music of Joni Mitchell. Victor was a couple of years younger than me.

Fortunately, there was a vegetarian café/restaurant adjacent to Pyramid called 'The Green Door' and as I was being paid what I thought at that time was generously, daily I got a take away from there of whichever salads they had made up and a slice of chocolate cheese cake if they'd made it. In the early days before the hostility was overt from Caroline the course co-ordinator who was recruited at the same time as me, we went to 'The Green Door' for a meal one lunch time. A couple of weeks earlier Cheryl and myself had been to the Brit Music Awards concert, and I harped on to Caroline about how sexy we'd found some of the artists, in particular James who performed his hit single 'All sit down'. She just nodded occasionally muttering "uhuh" completely disinterested, and kept her distance the whole time. It was when I'd finished my appraisal that I realized Caroline wasn't my only audience, but everyone else in the café had quietened down and was listening to what I was saying too. Caroline was a Christian who I overheard say to one of her friends in our office once that God spoke to her. I got the feeling that this was a regular occurrence. She'd also done a degree at the Laban Centre and had a dance troupe who use to rehearse at Pyramid. However like all of the other black girls I'd seen dance, contemporary dance that is, I felt they were all of them lacking in flexibility, suppleness, just as I had been. Those legs just didn't seem to want to fly in the way I'd seen them in white girls. Its not that I hadn't seen any good black dancers. I remember when I was doing O level dance at City and East London College, we went to see a performance of the Dance Theatre of Harlem, a troupe of

African-American ballet dancers from New York City. I was mesmerized by them.

January '91 I moved in with Cheryl. Her parents had bought the council house that they were living in and moved to Essex leaving the council house to Cheryl. Cheryl's youngest brother was living in Essex with his parents and her gay brother who was only a couple of years younger than her, was living with his partner elsewhere. In past conversations we'd had when we were both working at the CPS, Cheryl had told me her father was racist, so after I'd actually met him, I reminded her of that. She went up to her room and came down a couple of hours later. She told me she was really hurt by what I said and it had made her cry. Subsequently she denied that her father was racist. My move to Cheryl's place was partly the result of the discomfort I felt around my mum particularly as I was seeing Victor. I sensed her resentment when I stayed out overnight, or when I went out late. Gabriela on the other hand often turned up at my mums place all hours of the night to crash out, and all I saw from my mother toward her was adoration. In addition it was Cheryl that advised me to move out. In a telephone conversation I had with her during which we were discussing my fate she said pointedly, "I think you should get out of your mother's place," and that's exactly what I did.

I handed my assignment in to Plymouth, to keep my options open. When I left at the end of the second year, I was seriously considering not going back to finish my degree, but as nothing had changed for me apart from the location that I was in, I was beginning to reconsider. Anyway, while at Cheryl's place I bought for myself for the first time in my life, my very own TV, hi-fi, video and records. I selected my records carefully ensuring that most of the artists were of the African Diaspora. My memory for names in entertainment as well as the names of songs I like is very bad, so I took my cues from people at work and the papers in addition to flicking through the dance and soul sections of music shops.

One lunch time, I went to the Green Door to buy my lunch as usual and saw a black woman sitting outside as if she were waiting for someone. If I remember correctly, she followed me into the shop, and then started talking to me. She was African-American, and introduced herself as Nadine. Nadine Mnatzaganian. She was dark skinned, tall, exuberant, confident, bright and attractive. We exchanged numbers and in the following weeks, chatted on the phone quite often. She was in her mid thirties and was a Christian with the London Church of Christ. I went along to her church meetings which at the time were being held in the Odeon cinema in Leicester Square. I met her husband whom I was surprised to find was an English white man a few years younger than her. He was also one of the pastors in the church, and as such Nadine was a bible study leader, mentor and counsellor of the East London section of the church because they lived in East London. She was a qualified Educational Psychologist, although she was not currently working in the field. When I told her of my wishes to get into Clinical Psychology, she advised me strongly against it, saying it was an awful field to work in. Her position at the church afforded her many friends. Mostly black girls and women from what I could gather, and this fraternity of black women, made me want desperately to be a part of it because of the isolation I had felt from my experiences. Uppermost in my mind was a group of girlfriends I could go clubbing with and have girly chats with. Nadine however engineered the whole thing so that I didn't make friends of any of them and any time we were together, it was usually for a bible study. Reading from the bible one day she said, "I will make you a fisher among men," (from Matthew 4: 19 - 20) and then slightly amused quizzed me about being a fisher among men. Nadine had an incredible singing voice, just like the tradition of black female soul divas. When she sang the hymns in church, she reached all the high notes with the same volume as she did the low notes. I felt as though her voice could have reached *any* high note.

After church one Sunday, we sat in the MacDonald's restaurant Nadine crying and talking simultaneously. She was having a miscarriage and telling herself, "I'm being punished. It's because I took drugs when I was younger." She went on like this for some minutes, all the while crying. She invited me around to lunch too, with another friend of hers once. A white woman. Before her friend arrived, Nadine and I were having a discussion about men. She said that black men were haughty and the one thing she noticed about white men was that when they like black women, they liked them dark skinned. During lunch Nadine and her friend did most of the talking. Nadine's friend happened to mention that her husband was a policeman and I said with a derogatory tone, "I know all about the police." In one of my chats with Richard in the first year of being at poly, he told me he was picked up by the police once and beat up for no reason whatsoever. Although I didn't relay this to Nadine and her friend, I mentioned how unlawful and racist they were. Nadine's friend burst into tears, defending her husband, saying, "he was a good man."

Soon after starting work for Pyramid, I called Richard, and we arranged to meet in a pub in Bethnal Green. He looked good. Probably always had, but I just recognized it this time. Wearing a suit and grey coat, he looked the picture of success and made me feel quite cheap in comparison. As ever, he found the whole thing quite amusing, but plied me with complements anyway. He was working with computers, in what capacity I don't recall, but he'd bought a house in Willesden and was renting rooms out. Anyway, I was invited round to his place a couple of weeks later to see his house. It was the day on which Sophie and I went to the Black Hair and Beauty Show at the Business and Design Centre in Islington. Before we'd even arrived I spied two guys' one black and one white who looked like models. I perked up and harped on to Sophie about which one she thought was most attractive. As it happened, the pair of them were manning a stall on black skin products at the show and although I intentionally passed it by several times hoping to catch their attention, I never once plucked up the courage to speak to either of them. The show itself was great, particularly the fashion shows which included white models, even though I wondered what white models were doing at a Black Hair and Beauty Show? I mean, couldn't they find enough black models? I felt really sorry for the hostess of the fashion shows, a black girl who came out wearing an incredibly skimpy outfit, such that you could almost see her breasts. The crowd, full of black women started muttering 'slut' under their breath and dissing the hostess. Anyway, I admired all of the elaborate black hair do's I saw, but knew I wouldn't let the hair dressers touch my hair which was pulled back in a pony tail, even though I could have had it done for free on that day. So often I'd seen black girls get their hair done which always looked good initially, but after a few weeks would fall into a state barely resembling the original style. Not to mention what you had to do to look after it! Toward the end of the show, I left Sophie and made my way to Willesden.

It was quite late, and Richard was in by himself. His house was incredible. Apparently he'd gotten a huge bank loan with his cousin purchased the house and was in the process of renovating it. It had about seven or eight rooms and two bathrooms, one upstairs and one downstairs. There were carpets everywhere, and his room was like those you see in magazines. He had a double futon which was covered in a duvet with a black and white cover and a rug on the floor the same colour. There was a computer in one corner, a hi-fi and TV. We talked a little Richard being the first to introduce what I considered to be his girlfriend. A white woman a bit older than him whom he thought quite highly of, so I told him about Victor. I don't think either of us got any sleep that night. I left his place really early in the morning, as I was due at work that day and needed to clean up and change my clothes. I felt as though everyone knew what I'd been doing that night travelling back to Stratford on the underground in the morning. I felt so naked for some reason.

Apart from the fact that I felt inadequate and nervous at staff meetings, being at Pyramid Arts was a breeze. I was being paid more than I ever had been even though I didn't feel I deserved it and even though my self esteem was low,

I met a lot of interesting people. For Judith, the manager, Pyramid Arts Development was to be a dream in the making. She envisaged an arts centre in the heart of Hackney servicing in particular the local black community, like an arts centre she'd seen in Birmingham, that was run by black people. According to Judith Pyramid had a pretty controversial history which I didn't quite grasp the full story of. Basically it was previously run by a Rastafarian who was quite pally with the white people funding the project. I didn't quite understand why Judith said they liked him. Subsequently Pyramid received quite a bit of funding some of which was embezzled by the then staff. Anyway, management was then taken over by Jacob Ross who was also the manager or director of MAAS (Minority Arts Advisory Service) which was situated more or less down the road from Pyramid, and then management was passed on to Judith, who was dating Jacob Ross.

The general feeling held by management was that white people felt black people were incapable of running their own businesses, and Judith wanted to prove them wrong. Anyway it meant she had inherited a huge warehouse with three floors that needed vast amounts of funding to undergo a refurbishment programme before it even vaguely resembled a centre that people wanted to attend. One day Judith came to me and asked if I would attend a meeting at Shoreditch Town Hall that she'd completely forgotten about. It was regarding the future funding of arts projects in the voluntary sector. I was delighted to, as I felt I was simply required to sit and listen. However I was gravely mistaken. The meeting was an opportunity for arts projects in the voluntary sector to talk about how their project was servicing the community and why their project was so necessary. I think I was the only one who didn't say a word. I felt so frustrated. But worse than that was the fact that the man that led the discussion seemed to know who I was and indirectly consistently made digs at the fact that I hadn't said anything. He made references to lots of 'nervous projects' out there. In addition, there was a white guy there with a stammer who attempted speaking occasionally and when he did, he was encouraged by the people around him, as if they were trying to make a point. I felt as though through him, they were making an indirect reference to my situation. I froze. On returning from the meeting I was required to report back my feelings to Judith, which I did. I told her that basically, funding would be dependent on whether the organisation had a voice, and how adept your interpersonal skills were as it wouldn't hurt if you were able to massage the egos of those that were funding Pyramid. She seemed distressed at what I said.

On another occasion a white guy Dale McCrae, Pyramid's project manager from the London Borough of Hackney (all projects in the voluntary sector were required to have a representative from the local borough) arrived at Pyramid with a colleague to attend a meeting with Judith. As Judith wasn't immediately available they sat waiting for her in my office. While there, occasionally looking at me, he started talking about nervous breakdowns saying that some people didn't know when they were having them, and that you could have several, one after the other without knowing. I started to shake, and the more he spoke, the more nervous and frantic I became. Not only did I feel he was talking about me, but I started to wonder whether he was actually right even though I had heard or read literature that opposed this view. I felt perhaps I was delaying the inevitable, that in my stoic resistance to the innuendos wherever I went, my anxiety, the torment that accompanied the offences behind my back, my stammering and the nervous tic in my eye, that I should simply give up, and let it all 'hang out'. Go mad. But I couldn't do that because I wasn't insane. I had read or heard in a lecture that having a nervous breakdown was a loss of self control, and I clung on to that. I thought, no matter what happens, no matter how bizarre everything becomes, I just needed to stay in control.

The staff at Pyramid were divided. There were a few employees there who were present during the "good old days" when the Rastafarian was manager. It emerged one day while we were chatting in Victor's office that at least two of these employees, Chas and Duncan, felt as though Judith's intentions for Pyramid were dishonourable and she actually didn't want the project to succeed. I couldn't believe my ears. I know she didn't like me for whatever reason she had, but I also knew that she *was* genuine. Victor took the middle ground. Treated like a baby by the management and mentored by Judith, he was neither for nor against her.

One by one Victor's friends turned up at the office, and I was introduced to them. They all treated me highly respectfully. Niyi was a poet who had previously done a degree at university but didn't enjoy it at all. He recommended books for me to read regularly. He was thinking about doing an MA, but the thought of going back to university was too unbearable for him. In the same way that I couldn't explain to anyone what was happening to me, he didn't elaborate on why the thought of going back was so awful. Omari was mixed race, a vegan and very good looking. I thought to myself, where has he been hiding? It was only after Victor and I started dating that his friends started coming to the office. I thought if only I had been patient, maybe I could have been going out with Omari who wasn't as uncouth as Victor. Patrick arrived seemingly out of the blue one day too and offered his services to Victor. He was familiar with the music scene and I believe it was thought that his contacts would be useful. Another that made me regret my relationship with Victor. Patrick was trendy, wore his hair long in an afro with a trilby hat sat on top so that the rest stuck out at the sides. When he was in the office on his own I use to overhear him rapping, raps that he had created himself and he was good. Better than anything else I'd heard come out of Victor's office anyway. Patrick sang my praises to everyone and he was fascinated by my hair, its length and texture. He was dating a mixed race girl called Christine at the time. I assumed Victor had told him that we were going out with each other, but when I bumped into Patrick at the station one day and he kissed me on the lips telling me that we should meet up, I wondered what was going on. I asked him whether Victor had told him that we were going out with each other. He hadn't apparently, but as soon as Patrick heard, he backed off. Patrick was no stranger to attractive women. He was a DJ at various clubs, and I got the feeling girls poured themselves over him. He was certainly sure of himself.

It was Sophie who saw the advertisement in the Voice newspaper for a course in Black History. There and then we decided we would go. It wasn't the first time I'd thought about getting in touch with my roots. I went to the

African Cultural Centre in Dalston Lane when I was working at Sainsbury's and asked them if they did any Black History courses. They didn't, but the manager of the centre gave me a book by Basil Davidson called Africa In History which I found far too difficult to imbibe. Anyway the Black History course ran for about eight weeks. I met Lee Pinkerton there who was a good friend of Victor's too. He was currently working for MAAS as a journalist and had also previously done a degree at University. Once again I was taken aback by his looks, and wondered why I hadn't met him on my previous visit to the MAAS office. Going back from the class one evening, we wound up on the train together. His skin and body gleamed. I felt like a dried prune next to him. Both of us feeling a little awkward, he talked about his flat which he didn't like because it was in a tower block. I, desperate not to become any more of a stigma than I already was, talked about how nice the views were from tower blocks and that with a little decorating he could make it really appealing. He agreed with me eventually. The course itself made me wonder. I felt the teacher was vague and often resorted to sensationalism in his description of slavery. Maybe it really was awful, but something inside me niggled. What *really* happened back then? Anyway, at the end of the course I felt I was none the wiser about my roots.

It wasn't long after moving in with Cheryl that things between us started to deteriorate. Conversation became strained and Cheryl childishly became selfish with her knowledge. She stopped sharing her music and said she wanted to get into teaching and as a precursor to that wanted a lodger who was a teacher. There were three bedrooms in her house. She became the ice queen spitting her words out like the bullets from a machine gun when she spoke. Under these circumstances I invited her for a swim and sauna with me at the local baths. She said she hated swimming because she wasn't very good at it, but decided she'd come anyway. In the swimming pool, I was practically struggling to keep up with Cheryl. In the sauna I showed her the awful stretch marks I had on my backside. She said, "Everyone's got those," and showed me hers. Slight as she was, she had a few, not as bad as mine, but a few all the same. Cheryl was also a vegetarian and whereas the extra fibre from our diets seemed to congeal in my intestine, Cheryl was as regular as clockwork going several times in a morning. It was no wonder she was so slim. I discovered the more I eliminated, the slimmer were my hips and thighs so that having a bowel movement daily became almost an obsession for me. At about this time I bought some make-up too, but wasn't brave enough to wear it out. I was far too self conscious. I liked bright colours, pastels like blues, pinks and lilacs which I'd only ever seen white women wearing. And I remember when I was younger, occasionally I saw fat black women with blue eye shadow on and pink lipstick on their very full lips, and a white man by their side. I use to think they were prostitutes. Anyway I was sick of the dogma that I heard from both black and white people that only dark colours suited dark skins. Whereas white women could wear a range of colours from black through red to pink. So I took to wearing make-up around the house. I felt really special one day wearing sky blue eye shadow and a black 70's jump suit that had large purple flowers on it, a wrap around top half and was flared around the ankles. I think my mum bought it from a second hand market stall.

I went to Rainham to see Ricky one weekend who lived in a tower block. I told him nobody liked me. He said, "You're joking ain't ya?" He made me giggle. I thought about what it would be like to be Ricky's partner, both of us seeking enlightenment. There in his flat being so high up, it was really peaceful and everything was very tidy. I imagined life would be very simple and I was sure the negative experiences would come to an end, as if Ricky's spiritual power would somehow surround me with waves of positive energy that would influence the way people behaved toward me. I asked him what he did for sexual gratification, and he told me he masturbated. Without thinking about what I was doing, as if somnambulant, I asked him if he wanted to sleep with me. He declined. Ricky played the guitar well by ear and wanted to be a pop star. However, failing that he wanted to work in a bookshop that sold spiritual books. So that's what the social security office found for him, a job in a bookshop that sold spiritual books.

As a result of how guilty I felt about being at Pyramid, that is being paid and not having the communication skills to fulfil my role, I asked Judith if I could work part time. She would only have to pay me half the salary and I was sure I'd get done what was required of me. So, after a few months, I started working part time. In my days off at lunchtime, I went to the London Buddhist Centre in Bethnal Green and took part in the meditation classes. I also bought some B complex vitamin tablets as vitamin B was essential for good nervous functioning, and I thought they would stop the nervous tic in my eye. They didn't. I saw a counsellor once a week at Bodywise (which was affiliated to the London Buddhist Centre) in Bethnal

Green. When I went for my preliminary counselling
session, I discovered that my counsellor Martin Adams
also had a stutter. I wondered how he was going to counsel
me for a condition which he had himself. I was all ready to
end it there and then but he encouraged me to give him a
chance so I did. He also taught counselling skills at
Hackney Community College. Around Easter the London
Buddhist Centre were planning a weekend retreat. I signed
up for it, looking forward to what I considered to be a mini
vacation. I thought the people attending, mostly Buddhists
would be peaceable, and that I wouldn't have a lot to worry
about even though being cooped up with a bunch of
strangers left me slightly anxious about what I was going
to talk to them about. So we left one Friday night. About
twelve of us got into a van and were driven to the retreat by
a Scottish man who was also leading the whole weekend.
On arriving we all sat in a room and introduced ourselves.
There weren't enough seats for everyone to have one, so I
sat on the floor. Everyone sat against the walls, and I
found myself stuck alone in the middle feeling
uncomfortable at the stares that came my way. I was the
only black person present.

There was a fat man and his wife, who talked about his
exploits in Africa. He was an art dealer who sold African
artefacts. When *I* tried to say something he said, "We've
heard enough from you," and like a record that never ends,
continued talking. I found myself talking to a guy that
reminded me a lot of Perry. I think he said he was an
architect. Anyway I felt comfortable with him and we
chatted away for some time. At dinner that evening, I sat
next to him alongside two women. We talked about
holistic therapies and I chattered on about my experiences

at the Rainbow Centre. Then he asked me what a holistic therapy was. Although I didn't have a dictionary definition of it, I thought having participated in some therapies at the Rainbow Centre, I had a pretty good idea about it so I said, "Well it's a way of treating illness using alternative treatments and complementary medicine." The two women who sat near by half listening to our conversation in addition to talking amongst themselves turned to us and as though they were waiting for the opportunity to do this, like dogs going for the jugular said vociferously, "No it isn't! Its treatment that entails caring for the mind, body and soul!" Looking back on it, I think to myself well what's the big deal? I was partially right. But at the time I didn't rationalize it like that. Like a mute, I clammed up. The architect attempted to laugh it off, and continued talking with encouraging glances and nods in my direction but I just couldn't believe it was happening. The women seemingly glad of the opportunity to grab his attention filled my silence with conversation completely bypassing me as if I wasn't there. There I was on a Buddhist retreat hoping to have my nerves soothed and to forget about the distressing circumstances of my life, and it seemed that that was impossible. There was no escape. The weekend was going to be a nightmare.

I don't know how I got through the rest of the weekend, I avoided everyone as much as possible. I was sharing a bedroom with two others, one of the women saying she was a black belt in karate. Another of the women went round humming to herself the whole time. My skin tingled and my eyes stung I was so tense. I attempted to console myself on the Saturday by washing my hair as if that were going to make everything better. I didn't sleep a wink the whole weekend. The others, in between meditation sessions, went for walks and cooked the meals together. When we got back to London I said goodbye to everyone and the Scottish man looking at me intently said quite solemnly, "Take good care of yourself." Shortly after arriving back at Cheryl's place she had a short phone call during which she didn't say very much. But, when she put the phone down she said half to me and half to herself, "You're in trouble Rosie Mitchell." I was so exhausted from the weekend and ready for the unexpected, that I didn't even bother asking her what she meant. I simply went up to my room, shut the door, collapsed on the bed and cried.

Still determined to make a go of things, I enrolled for some evening classes. The only one which proved to be successful socially was a Latin American Dance Class at the Tom Allen Theatre in Stratford. There were only a handful of people at the class, among them two young men, who weren't being discreet about their thoughts of me. They nudged and whispered to each other. I overheard one of them say, "Look at her a**e!" They made me feel uncomfortable, but not in a nasty way. At the end of the class I was invited to join them for a drink. They introduced themselves as Peter and Stuart. Peter was Ghanaian, and Stuart was half Indian and half white. I was nervous, but they were so friendly, I was able to share that with them. I accepted an offer of a cigarette and something to drink, all the while my nerves so evident you could see my hands shaking. They found it amusing. And that was the beginning of our friendship. They were both a few years younger than me, and as the weeks went by I realized that they weren't as pally with each other as they appeared.

They met at the dance class, and they were actually quite different. Stuart was in his second year at East London Polytechnic doing a Cultural Studies degree and Peter was working and still living at home with his mother.

Occasionally I met with Gabriela or Jessica who were even more frequent clubbers than myself, mainly because their social circumstances allowed it. Before the tension began to build up from Cheryl toward myself we went out with Gabriela and her friends to the Shenola night club back then off Carpenter's Lane, a regular haunt of Gabriela's. Days before going we asked Gabriela what sort of thing we should wear, to which she replied more or less anything. So one weekend, dressed pretty much in jeans and shirt we met up with Gabriela, Aisha and Denise, all of whom were dressed up to the nines. Inside, the club was full of women in figure hugging, short, smart clothes, not to mention the men. Not only that, but a white girl in Shenola's? To say the least we felt uncomfortable. To top it all the music wasn't the upbeat dance hits of the very early 90's which had mostly black composers, but mainly ragga which I disliked terribly. Disappointed, we left early leaving Gabriela and her friends behind, Cheryl commenting that it would have helped if we were given sound advice about the dress code. Sheepishly I agreed. There was another incident when Gabriela's seeming self-centredness was brought to the fore. Working for Islington Council she harped on about her boss to me, telling me that she thought we would get on really well. She talked about him so much that I even began to believe her as her description of him reminded me a lot of Perry. So when the opportunity came up to go to the theatre and meet with him, I agreed. Her work place were arranging a day out to see 'Five Guys

Named Mo.' The tickets were between £20 and £30, so I paid her my money and arranged to meet her at Bethnal Green Station one Saturday afternoon where we were going to make our way to the theatre together. I waited well over one hour at the arranged time and when there was no sign of Gabriela I contemplated going to the theatre alone, but as I didn't know who her work mates were (and they held the tickets), I went home, furious. I think I managed to catch up with her on the phone the following day. When I asked her what happened she said she'd been visiting Junior her boyfriend who was in prison for burglary outside of London. She said it couldn't be helped. So I asked her for my money back and she said as though I were the one being ridiculous, "You're not getting it!" She proceeded to justify why I wasn't getting my money back and I became more and more wound up. It wasn't that I needed the money, it was just her whole attitude about the situation. She acted as though she were in the right. It was a while after, a few months perhaps, that eventually she came to her senses and apologized, and gave me back my money.

At around this time Gabriela bought a house in East Ham with a friend of her mothers' called Gene. The arrangement between them was that Gabriela gave Gene the money each month to pay her half of the mortgage, but after a while, Gene stopped paying it and kept it for herself. Not long after, Gabriela got letters from the bank threatening her with repossession of the house. She moved out a year or so later, and when she was 22 years old, bought a flat of her own. I wanted my own house too. I couldn't bare to live in what I considered to be the mayhem of my mother's abode, and sharing accommodation wasn't proving to be too hot either. Not only that, but Gabriela was five years my junior, and there she was settling down already. The thought of having my own space, and not having to put up with the whims of others was really appealing to me, but there was no way I was able to afford a place of my own on my salary. I attempted to solicit the assistance of my niece Jessica, suggesting that we could buy a place together, as I knew that she was also having problems with the people she was sharing accommodation with. She flatly refused and gave me the impression that she felt I would be the sole benefactor. Her reasoning baffled me to say the least.

Desperate for friendship, I applied to ads in lonely hearts columns. I simply felt as though I was suppose to be having the time of my life. After all, I was young. I had two encounters from this venture. One was with a white guy who I met in a pub in Hampstead Heath. We went walking on the heath, and nothing came of our relationship, but I was keen to know what his impression of me was because I was permanently stunned by everyone's seeming dislike of me. He said he was going through a therapy called Re-birthing that entailed as the name suggests being born again. I didn't try to understand what you were reborn as or how the re-birthing experience came about, because at that time, I wasn't interested. My second encounter was with a black lesbian girl called Rosie. This relationship lasted a little bit longer although it was awkward at times. She was convinced that I was a lesbian so eventually, shopping in Central London one day with Rosie in a foul mood for some reason, we just drifted apart. We didn't even say goodbye. However during our friendship, we went to the women's night at the Fridge nightclub in Brixton where I met her gay girlfriends, and on one occasion we met up with Jessica to see a play at the Hackney Empire.

Everything that happened was tinged with adversity. Jessica and I went to the Camden Palace one night, and while we were standing in the queue to get in there were two white men behind us not typical of the crowd at the club. One said to the other while looking at Jessica and myself, "Some of us are developing interesting personalities these days aren't we?" Jessica nudged me and whispered, "Did you hear what they said?" I told her I had, and in the same breath told her to ignore them. But I was afraid. It was another addition to the innuendos that followed me wherever I went, and didn't understand why. Jessica was a lot more aggressive than me, and it was for this reason that I invited her back to Cheryl's place one evening. I wasn't afraid of Cheryl exactly, but she had me on edge all of the time. I couldn't match the short, sharpness she adopted in conversation with me in the latter half of our relationship. So we three sat around the kitchen table chatting, and as if by magic Cheryl fumbled and got nervous although she still had verbal diarrhoea. Jessica took it all in her stride slowly and patronizingly saying things like, "Could you repeat what you just said?" "Now, really Cheryl?" I often wondered why I didn't have that effect on people. But Jessica's circumstances were not all a bed of roses. I was never sure what was going on exactly. We met in a pub by Highbury and Islington station one day and it was quite crowded. We chattered about this and that and I said half jokingly and half serious, "How's you're love life?" Jessica mumbled something that was incoherent and then excused herself to go to the loo.

When she got back she said threateningly, "Don't you ever ask me about my personal affairs again!" I was taken aback, but saw that she was serious. There were gasps and remarks of "Ooh!" from the crowd at the table adjacent to us. They had been listening to our conversation.

At Pyramid, Victor was releasing a record. It was hardcore rap and I told him it was rubbish and it wouldn't get anywhere. I mean I was no connoisseur of music, but I think I knew a good song when I heard one, not that my taste in music necessarily had any impact on the hits that got in the charts. Anyway he fussed about the sleeve cover deciding on the typical icons of rap music i.e. girls and cars. He asked Caroline if her dance group would be interested in participating in a photo shoot, completely bypassing me. He'd get together with his friends, and excitedly brag about how it was going to be. Likewise Caroline's dancers often congregated in our office in an excited but contained hype. It wasn't only this incident that led me to the following conclusion, but Victor didn't value me. I felt he was totally self-centred. After hearing some of the music that he listened to, I decided that his disregard of me was an attitude he held of all women, influenced in particular by his liking for rap music. There was an African accountant at Pyramid too called Steve Nartey who I spent quite a bit of time with because he was affable and mild mannered. He hit on me a couple of times, after which I stopped spending time with him because I thought he obviously misread the situation. It wasn't long after that I saw extremely attractive African women coming to see him at Pyramid as if he were showing me what for. Sitting at the reception area one day a close friend of Betty's walked in (Betty being the girl who warned me about being too clever in my first year of being at Plymouth). She said she hadn't seen Betty in a long time and she was wondering what had happened to her. It seemed she had simply disappeared.

Tania was the only one from my school friends who I kept in touch with. After doing a foundation year at Camberwell Art College, she did a degree at Farnham Art College in Surrey and then went on to do an MA at the Royal College of Art in London. I was invited to her house share in Farnham on a couple of occasions. Once for a party she gave before I went to Plymouth and again simply for a break at the weekend in my year out. She shared with among others two girls, Nay and Kim, who were not twins but dressed identically, and who were both very slim with blonde hair. They were the belles of the ball at the party Tania had invited me to, but on the second occasion I met them, they took an instant disliking of me. I'm not sure why. Tania almost worshipped them, and I wondered whether it was anything she had said to them about me. Back at Cheryl's place, my discomfort increased quite severely, particularly when Cheryl's dream of having a teacher move in was fulfilled. The teacher was an Indian woman called Anita, originally from Leicester I think it was. Cheryl was in her elements. Anita was loud and completely uninhibited, and both she and Cheryl got on like a house on fire. I tried to build a rapport with Anita, but I simply wasn't quick enough and to top it all, I didn't have any positive experiences to talk about. Cheryl and Anita liked the same programmes, talked about the TV show hosts and presenters as if they were their neighbours and laughed a lot, but whenever I walked into the room they fell silent. In spite of these circumstances, still not having learned my lesson, I went out clubbing with them on a couple of occasions. I suppose I was still trying to forge some feeling of happiness. Of course I would come home feeling more miserable than before the evening began. Typically Cheryl and Anita talked and giggled with each other as though I wasn't there, and me feeling like a lemon would do my best to look as though I were having a good time.

I spent more and more time in my room, my resentment for Cheryl building, and wanting desperately to avenge her of her hostility toward me. Well the opportunity came up once. I planned an evening out with Maria (the girl I met in Plymouth) and Cheryl. Before the night out I explained the situation about Cheryl and myself to Maria and I told Maria that when we were out she was to completely ignore Cheryl. I wanted Cheryl to feel how she made me feel when she was with Anita. So that's what we did. Whenever Cheryl said something I completely ignored her and did my best to keep the conversation flowing between Maria and myself as though she wasn't there. My feelings while doing this were conflicting. I felt so bad, and nervous, but at the same time it felt good. But this planned revenge didn't last very long. A guy, long haired hippy type, walked over to Cheryl and started to chat her up. I couldn't believe her luck. On my 24th birthday, I'd arranged to go out for a meal and then on to the Wag night club in Wardour Street. I invited Gabriela and her friend, Paul, Stuart and stupidly, caught up in the excitement of it all, Cheryl. I had previously told Cheryl that I liked Stuart, but it didn't stop her from making a bee line for him the whole evening. I didn't have anything to worry about though, he simply wasn't interested, although I felt they would have made a good couple. They were both intelligent, knowledgeable and sharp.

I started looking for alternative accommodation shortly after. I found a room in a house that was just across the road from West Ham Park in Caistor Park Road. There was one black girl living there who was a nurse called Margaret, and a younger white girl who occupied one of the rooms downstairs. She was going out with a black guy. After seeing Margaret I thought I couldn't let this opportunity pass me by. I was sure that we could become good friends. We didn't. She kept herself to herself but at least I'd seen an end to the antics at Cheryl's place. The house stunk to high heaven when I first moved in. It smelled of a smell resembling lard that I associated with white people. It was disgusting, so for the first few weeks I left the windows open, and thoroughly hoovered and cleaned all of the communal areas in addition to my room. There was a garden, but it looked as though it hadn't been attended to for years and the kitchen and dining room that were adjacent to the garden at the back of the house downstairs were crawling with woodlice. It made my skin crawl, but as my bedroom was upstairs, I overlooked it thinking I should consider myself lucky anyway. My landlords were policeman who were surprisingly really nice. Both quite young, late twenties early thirties, and the rent was cheap. When I told Judith at work that I had moved house, she said laughing, "They say the best way to lose a friend is to move in with them."

I went jogging a couple of times a week, and in my days off I went to the park and finding a dog dirt free spot which was almost impossible, I sunbathed. Victor came over occasionally when I would rent a video, usually of black interest, cook lots to eat and we would just hang out in my room. Richard came over once or twice too. I remember an occasion when he phoned up out of the blue one evening saying he wanted to come over. I think it was a Sunday. Anyway, like a headless chicken I rushed around trying to get hold of some condoms. I knew *he* wouldn't have any, even though I also knew sex would be on the agenda. There was also Stuart. Such was my admiration for his intellect, that when he asked me out I consented, even though I was going out with Victor. Stuart was like a teenager from an American movie. We would go over to West Ham park and monkey-like he would play the fool, hanging from the climbing frames wise cracks like champagne from a recently opened bottle spilling out of him. He made me feel like I was a world away even though I could barely match his wit. Stuart was one of those guys who liked most things about black culture. He was a fan of the music of Dina Caroll, and introduced me to the rap group De La Soul. He even put grease in his hair, much to my amazement. Stuart and I bumped into Niyi while we were on our way to the mall in Stratford one day. I had bought a video that wasn't working properly, and I had asked Stuart if he would give me a lift to the mall. The video machine was quite heavy. To ease the guilt I felt at using Stuart as a mini cab service, I told him I would carry the video to the shop once we were out of the car. It was at this point that we saw Niyi, me struggling with the video machine and Stuart walking by my side. Niyi followed us into the shop before introducing himself, and then he gave Stuart an extremely dirty look which judging from Stuart's excitement at meeting a black brother, he hadn't noticed. When Stuart and I were out together, we were stared at by black men, and once while playing tennis a group of black guys walked past the tennis courts whispering to each other and shouting, "Slut!" At the time, I thought they were spies of Victor's. It didn't make me feel guilty though as I was sure Victor was seeing other women. I caught him flirting with a girl once on the way to work. She looked all ragged and tarty like a prostitute, and I wondered whether they'd spent the night together. I thought to myself, he wouldn't know if she were a prostitute if it were written across her forehead. Not only that, but when he got a car he refused to take me for a drive in it and he would harp on about the adventures him and his friends had driving around London.

One evening I suggested to Stuart that we drive over to see my niece Jessica. She wasn't on the phone, so I couldn't tell her we were coming, but I thought it would be nice, and that we could all spend the evening together. So in his father's car, Stuart drove us over to Stoke Newington. When we got to Jessica's place, we were let in by one of her house mates. We made our way up to the top floor which is where her room was, knocked on the door and went in. Jessica was in her dressing gown, and as if she had been in a tussle with someone, the room looked like a bomb had hit it. Furniture had been overturned, the bed was unmade, and everything was generally dishevelled. As I looked around taking it in she simply said, "Yep." I wasn't sure what had taken place in her room that day and remembering the time I asked her about her love life in the pub, I was sure asking would simply have made her agitated. So I said, "I guess you're not ready for visitors just now," and after a very short conversation with her, Stuart and I left. I had been round to Jessica's place a couple of months earlier too. I cycled over after work one evening. I remember her looking terribly thin, but I was determined not to make an issue of it, because I thought I was projecting, that is, I thought I would have been voicing *my* concerns about food from my compulsive eater days. She was overcome by excitement, thrilled it would seem by a new man in her life. As was usual for us whenever we visited each other, I asked her what she had for me to eat, and while she chit chatted about problems with the house share, her new lover and family, I ate smoked mackerel with salad. We didn't see each other for a while after that. Not until I was back at Poly anyway.

Stuart and I didn't last very long. We never actually had sex, and one evening when I was at his place, I said I thought it would be best if we call it quits. We remained good friends though, for a while anyway.

I continued meeting up with Nadine for church on Sundays, and it was her that prompted me to ask Victor for commitment. I don't know what gave her the impression he wasn't committed. I don't recall saying much to her about our relationship. So just before I was due to go back to Poly (oh by the way I decided to go back as being at Pyramid didn't give me any cause to hope) I confronted Victor about commitment. Not marriage or anything like that, just confirmation that we would be faithful to each other. He dillied and dallied and as if I were trying to catch hold of a live fish, he twisted everything I said and refused to commit himself. So I said, "I suppose we'd better say goodbye then?" and he did. Of course, I cried in my room afterward. I was frightened to go back to

Plymouth, and it would have been comforting to know that there was someone waiting for me, back in London.

I was trying to open myself up to the idea of God in the Christian sense. Spirituality, had failed me. The peace that I expected when I embarked on my spiritual journey simply hadn't happened. I knew that my ego (what I had of an ego anyway) had to be crushed if I were going to achieve enlightenment, but I simply hadn't expected it quite to follow the circumstances that had taken place in my life since taking on that philosophy. If the change in my life circumstances were what spirituality had to offer, then I didn't want it. So I read the bible, not really understanding what I was reading, but with the faint hope that God would protect me. My brother Payton called me about this time, telling me that Terrence who was then living somewhere in Tottenham was having a spot of trouble. We went over to his place to see what the problem was. Both he and his partner Joanne told us the same thing. They said their TV switched channels by itself and sometimes when they arrived back home from being out, evil messages were scrawled on their bedroom mirror in lipstick. Neither of them appeared terribly frightened and certainly at least at that time, I was of the belief that everything had a rational explanation. I thought they were lying to us, but I couldn't work out why. They were both unemployed, and spent most of their time watching horror movies. They even suggested we turn on the TV and witness it changing channels by itself. So I confiscated the remote controls to both the TV and the video and we turned on the TV. Nothing happened. They were both looking quite desperate, so I suggested that I say a prayer, and read from the bible. I was frightened. Terrence had earned himself a reputation in some extremely violent fights, and I wasn't sure what he was capable of. So standing at the opposite end of the room to him, I said a prayer, and read from the bible.

When my brother and I left, we went to the local Catholic church and asked the priest if they would pay Terrence a visit. Whether he did or not, I'm not sure, but we didn't hear any more about any strange occurrences from Terrence and Joanne.

At about this time, at home one afternoon, I received a phone call from Maria's brother. He asked me if I was one of Maria's friends and then proceeded to tell me that Maria had committed suicide. She had taken an overdose of the pills she was taking. Her brother told me where the funeral was being held if I was interested in attending and that was the last I heard of Maria. I was pretty shocked. I wonder what drove her to suicide in the end. She told me she was living in a hostel run by MIND and the guy in the room next door to hers was driving her insane because he played his music so loudly, but who knows.

Sophie and I remained good friends throughout this period, and with Cheryl off of the scene, I spent more and more time with her. One night alongside her cousins and friends we arranged to go to Trends nightclub that was then off of Dalston Lane in Roseberry Place. I had arranged to meet Sophie at Liverpool Street station, and as I was running late waiting for the bus, I decided to hitch a lift. An Asian guy pulled up in a really smart white car across the road and went into the chip shop. I went over to him, and bold as brass, asked him for a lift to Liverpool street station.

Surprisingly he consented and away we went. When we got into the city he went down a one way street against the flow of traffic, not intentionally. Neither of us knew our way around. Anyway, there was none other than the traffic police waiting around the corner and he was hailed to one side. I felt so sorry for him, but thanked him for the lift, told him I was late and then rushed off. As it happened, Sophie and her friends were late anyway, so I found myself waiting outside Liverpool street station. When they finally arrived, I found they were all wearing mini skirts. They had obviously consulted each other about this before hand, and I felt disheartened that I hadn't been involved. I was wearing a pair of grey pegs and black blouse that had a square neck line revealing the upper part of my chest. The club wasn't that great, for me anyway. I wasn't that keen on the music which everyone else seemed to love. I was more into the dance music of that era which was then a combination of styles. There was a modelling competition on at the club that night and Sophie encouraged me to enter. She said that I could go up on the stage and loosen my hair from its pony tail and shake it out, believing I was bound to win. I thought about my glasses, which I believe were the national health styled ones at that time and looked around at the unrestrained crowd and decided against it. I was sure they would boo me off.

Back at the house, the ceiling in the dining room had cracks in it which I pointed out to one of the landlords one evening when he was checking up on us. I told him that he'd better do something about it, because it was bound to cave in. He said it would be fine. We often had problems in the bathroom too, which was directly above the dining room. The hot water was always cutting out, and as a result I would have to have cold showers. I can't remember why I wasn't keen on filling the sink in the bathroom from the kettle, but I wasn't. On one of my days off, I'd arranged to meet Sophie at her cousins place where we were going to spend the day watching videos and eating. Lo and behold, I went downstairs to make some breakfast and saw that the dining room ceiling had caved in and water was pouring down. I didn't have a clue where the stop-cock was and as we couldn't use the telephone to make outgoing calls, I had to make my way to a phone box to call the landlords. Their answering machine was on so I left a message for them to call me urgently at the house. They were pretty annoyed that I didn't know where the stop-cock was but when they told me (beneath the floor boards just before the front door) I switched the water off not having washed, and went on my way to meet Sophie.

It was sweltering outside, not that I was complaining. I loved the sun. However, I was feeling a little grubby, as I hadn't washed that morning. When I arrived at Sophie's cousins place, we got some videos and snacks and sat around in the living room chatting for a while. I handed some leaflets out that I had obtained from a fortnightly meeting at Brixton Town Hall on prominent figures/issues in the black community. No one seemed interested. Anyhow, wafts of my body odour kept infusing my nostrils, and it wasn't long before everyone subtly moved away from me. Whenever I moved closer to them, they moved again. I started to get really nervous, so excused myself to go to the bathroom where I thought I'd be able to wash up a bit. It was awful. I felt like a traveller. Anyway there wasn't a towel to be found in the bathroom much less soap. Perhaps they kept their things in their rooms because it was shared accommodation. A couple of minutes later I went back into the living room and everyone went quiet as if they knew what I went into the bathroom for. Zenna's brother smiled at me, I smiled at him and we both started laughing as if the whole thing was a big joke. He was the only one that made me feel normal that day. We got chatting, and it wasn't long before my body odour no longer seemed the centre of attention, thankfully.

Ruth, got married at around this time and I was invited to both the hen night and the wedding. Ruth's husband to be was at her hen night with one of his friends either because he'd travelled so far away from his home that none of his friends could make his stag night or because, if I recall correctly, Ruth said something about him not having any friends. I'm not entirely sure which was true. I hadn't been to many weddings, only one other when I was in my teens, my sister Claudia's wedding, so I wasn't that well acquainted with wedding etiquette. Suffice it to say, I didn't buy anything new for the occasion. I wore a flowery dress that I liked, but that had been worn on numerous previous occasions. I was a touch embarrassed when I saw how well everyone else had turned up. I invited Peter to come along with me. He turned up dressed in quite a smart suit. We were late for the church service, but met all my old school pals at the reception afterwards that was held in a pizzeria on Bethnal Green Road that I had been to on numerous previous occasions. I didn't see much of Ruth throughout the whole occasion. There was some resentment from Jackie Fearon towards me. She antagonized everything I said. Not sure what I did to deserve that, but otherwise the whole occasion passed extremely smoothly. Peter and I jumped at the opportunity to show off our salsa dance skills when the song 'Lambada' came on. Everyone was impressed. Half way through Ruth and her husband were whisked away to their honeymoon, leaving the rest of us to pick at the buffet that had been spread especially for the occasion.

Toward the end of the summer, my thoughts returned to Plymouth. I was scared to go back. Not only that but I had to think about what I was going to do for my final year project. I wanted to do something that was going to maintain my interest, something that wouldn't be a bind to research. The few ideas I had, involved subjects of problems that I encountered in my life, the main one being differences in communicative ability between humanities/social science students and science students. As a BSc Psychology student, I classified myself as a science student. My course was more science than arts based as I was told it was the BSc that opened you up to more job opportunities. We were often told by the lecturers that psychology was desperately trying to become recognized as a pure science as it is only with this status that the research that arose from the subject would be valued. Anyway, I lapped up the contents of the course that were more concerned with personal psychology, philosophy, social psychology, the more arts based contents of the subject. If I were true to myself, I should definitely have been on a BA rather than BSc, but at that time there was only one BA Psychology course in the whole of the UK, and that was based at Sussex University which I hadn't even applied to. But my concern about communicative ability was that humanities/social science students seemed to be more articulate than science students and I wanted to prove firstly whether this was true, and second, why (if it were true) this was the case. It was clear to me, that the more articulate you were, the more contented you were, and the more likely you were to be successful.

Just before I returned to Plymouth Spike Lee's movie Jungle Fever came out. I was excited about it as I was with all of Spike Lee's movies at that time. Peter and I made an occasion of going to see it. We set a day aside and went into Central London. It was after the movie that Peter suggest I use the themes prevalent in it for my final year project.   Overwhelmed with excitement I decided the subject of my study would be 'interracial attraction' although I had no idea what shape or form it would take. My initial idea was that I would show both black and white people pictures of 'attractive' black and white people and get them to rate them on attractiveness. My theory was that both groups of subjects would rate the pictures of white people as being more attractive. However I envisaged all sorts of problems with a study of this kind. First and foremost, I had to find a set of pictures of black and white people which had an equal rating of attractiveness. It was a subject that I was passionate about though, and it was certainly going to maintain my interest.

At Pyramid, I wound my appointment to a conclusion. Gave in my notice, and told Judith I had decided to go back to Plymouth to finish my degree. I was encouraged by one of the committee members called Carmen who incidentally was also on the interviewing panel. She told me I was doing the right thing, and that there was nothing for me at Pyramid grimacing when she mentioned the Art Centre's name. In the six months that I had been there, not one bit of refurbishment had been carried out. The programme was extensive and expensive and it was proving near impossible to attract funding to complete it. Employing the architects it seemed had been a complete waste of time and money because not one of their plans had been put into effect.

While I was living with Cheryl, I had undergone some drugs counselling training, an opportunity I thought to gain some experience in counselling. The idea was given to me by Man Yee and Gemma who joined 'Nightline' a phone counselling service for distressed students, in their second year at Plymouth. At that time I was more like one of the students needing counselling rather than attempting to add to my work skills, so I didn't even think about it. The truth is, not much had changed for me since being at Plymouth, but I felt if I ploughed on, even if I wasn't enjoying it, the horrible situation I found myself in would come to an end. During the training itself I was once again flooded by everyone's apparent brilliance. Most, if not all, it seemed had keen minds, and it all left me wondering once again what happened to me. I decided I disliked the training tutor when the one other black person on the course, a black man, went to say something, and he was interrupted by the tutor. I felt it was tough enough for black people without the insensitivity the tutor demonstrated in that moment. Be that as it may, I finished the training and at the end of the summer had one sessions worth of experience at East London Drugs Project, then in Bethnal Green, where I was sure the co-ordinator of the project, an ex-junkie, was still on drugs he was so quick and shook constantly. After that, I was all set for Plymouth.

Chapter 10: Plymouth Again

Stuart agreed to drive me to Plymouth a few days before
the beginning of term so that I would have enough time to
look for accommodation. In my first year at poly there
were rumours about the allocation of halls to freshers.
Apparently, they had allocated the dilapidated halls that
were further away from the polytechnic to working class
students, and the newer more modern halls on the doorstep
of the polytechnic, to middle class students. I wondered
whether the experience of my first two years had
prejudiced them against me and they had me blacklisted in
their files. It was Cheryl who alerted me to the idea of
individuals being blacklisted by organisations. Back then,
she was referring to the civil service. I felt, as I did with
most of Cheryl's gloomy thoughts, that she was being
paranoid, and yet there I was, an incarnation of her
pessimism.

When we arrived in Plymouth, we went straight to the
accommodation office where I was handed one address, a
house share with five or six students. If I remember
correctly, it was late afternoon. We made our way to the
address and was invited in by a plump girl. She showed
me into the living room which was nothing special, but
reminded me of my mother's place. It had a lived in feel
about it. The furniture covers, wallpaper and carpets were
slightly faded, and there were a few plants dotted around
the room. Then she showed me up to the available room.
It was at the top of the house. I wasn't expecting a palace,
but I most definitely was not expecting a cat's litter tray
either. Dotted around on the carpet at various stages of
decay was cat's pooh. She said grinning, as if it were

amusing, "This is the room," and mentioned something about cleaning the cat's pooh up if I were interested. I didn't know what to say so I looked around the room pretending to take in its features as though I were considering taking it. The truth was like an indelible stain, images of the cats pooh flooded my mind, and I had already decided that I wasn't taking the room. As if she heard my thoughts, she said, "There is another room, but it's a lot smaller than this one. Would you like to see it?" I said that I would and just across the landing we made our way to the other room which was like a matchbox, but cat pooh free. She left us then for a while telling me that I could think about it and let her know what I had decided. When she left the room, I told Stuart that there was no way I was taking either room. As if it were his house, he attempted to coax me into settling for the matchbox sized room commenting that the first was dodgy, but this one seemed alright. I suppose he just wanted to go home. By that time the accommodation office was closed, so I couldn't check out any more rooms that evening. I told him I would go back to the accommodation office first thing in the morning. We told the girl that showed us the room that I was undecided, but if anything I would settle for the smaller of the two rooms. She allowed us to stay the night.

So, we had an evening to fill together in Plymouth. I attempted to act as though I were the typical student, lots of friends, nights out at the student union, happy. Who was I trying to kid? I took Stuart to see long haired Steve and Mike both of whom had also taken a year out and were sharing a flat not far from the poly. Steve was his usual cynical self, hinting at my experience in the second year.

Mike was more diplomatic. My attempts to steer my way through this verbal minefield, already had me running away mentally if not physically. Stuart I felt, sensed the tension, but like the witty student he was, coolly played it off as though it were just another social gathering. Anyway, I asked them if they wanted to join us at the student union. They declined, so Stuart and I said our goodbyes, and made our way to the poly.

The student's union was teeming with students and for a while I felt excited. That was until the carry on behind me began. Surrounded by students, I stood talking to Stuart, and then I sensed someone did something behind my back so that Stuart witnessed it. Like everyone else, he said nothing, leaving the turmoil within me to boil. Too afraid to turn around and call their bluff just in case they confidently confirmed my thoughts about my teetering sanity and ashamed by the fact that a large number of students witnessed this insidious slight against me and instead of wondering why it was happening, feeling sorry and perhaps trying to make amends (like I would) joined in with the persecution mainly by remaining silent, I too remained silent. We left shortly after, and on the way back to the house where we were staying Stuart distant and cloaked with a look that I felt was apprehension he expressed his gratitude that he was at East London Polytechnic the incident at the student union remaining unspoken of between us. As I did with all of my so called friends whom I felt let me down regarding this carry on, I contemplated terminating our friendship but then thought better of it. I was too desperate to be friendless.

The following morning, we made our way to the accommodation office. I told them the address they had given me the previous day was unsuitable so they punched me into the computer again, and churned out another address. When we arrived at the house in Roseberry Avenue, St Judes, the door was answered by a young guy in decorating overalls. He invited us in where we found he was painting the walls in the back yard. The house was spic span and a definite improvement on the last place we saw. I allowed Stuart to do most of the talking, even though it was me that was moving in. I was a nervous wreck, you see Mark was very well spoken and this made me even more anxious. Maybe it was a combination of being in Plymouth and the fact that he was a student that brought this on, but once again I found myself unable to function. Stuart pulled me aside and asked me what I thought, and I said I couldn't cope. Stuart, as though he'd spent a lifetime mingling with Mark types and probably had, assured me that Mark was alright. For some reason I then thought that Stuart perceived Mark as a nerd, which is why he wasn't threatened by him, and this realization calmed me down a little. When Mark showed us to the vacant room, my wits about me again I chatted a little. The house felt comfortable. The room was large and clean and even though it was a little way from the polytechnic, I decided to take it. The rent was cheap too.

We unloaded my stuff from Stuart's car, then I said my goodbyes to Stuart and I was on my own. Leaving my bedroom door open, I fixed my belongings in my room and then oiling my legs, was interrupted by Darryl who was on the same course as Mark and had the room to the right of mine. I felt comfortable engaged in this occupation (oiling my legs) with a male student as I felt less was expected of me by way of conversational gymnastics. Darryl was nice enough and with our introduction over, I decided I was going to get some shopping. Mark offered to give me a lift to Sainsbury's on his motorbike. I had to undo my pony tail to get the helmet on, and once we were outside Sainsbury's taking the helmet off, I had an image of my hair falling down about my shoulders like you see in adverts. Instead, it hung stiffly in one clump at the back of my head, and when Mark had left, I wondered whether I had gotten grease on the inside of his helmet. After getting my shopping, I got a cab back to my new home. Geoff, an African guy from London moved in a few days later occupying the box room to the left of mine. He was doing a degree in computing studies and remembering something Janet said from my second year (that all I needed was a boyfriend and everything would look a lot better for me) I considered flirting with him to see if I could get him to go out with me. When I tried, I felt as though he knew exactly what I was up to and he kept bursting into giggles. I didn't think I could sink much lower. He wasn't intellectual at all and wore a wide dumb grin whenever I saw him

Being at the poly was as I expected. I was tense, and nervous. During my first meeting with my tutor Dave Rose, I attempted to open up to him about my anxiety at being in Plymouth again. He cut me short saying that I had better be good as he was responsible for my references, so I avoided him for the rest of the year. I had been placed in some interesting course options for my final year. Among them was group behaviour in social psychology that was being taught by Dr Fraser Reid. In all lectures began the tireless innuendos that I had become accustomed to. This was particularly true in Fraser Reid's lectures who I felt was telling me indirectly that I had his support. Not surprisingly, I took a liking to him. He looked blonder than I had remembered him from my first two years, and he was well built. Not only that, but he was the most eloquent lecturer that I had come across, and this I found extremely attractive.

It wasn't long before the carry on started behind my back. Whenever I was out wherever I was whether it was around the poly or in Plymouth City Centre people standing behind me did things at me. This led to the typical pattern of emotions that I had become accustomed to although this didn't make it any easier to deal with. Due to the fact that people were talking about me in my first two years, I was more or less friendless, so I held everyone at arms length too ashamed and afraid to ask anyone why this was happening to me, just in case they implied I was mad. I was fragile as it was. I decided it was better to put up with everybody's pretence that everything was ok rather than rumours or glances that implied I was losing it. My dandruff didn't help the situation any. I had taken to washing my hair as frequently as possible, once every two weeks, which I felt was as much as my hair could take before it started breaking and falling out. But in between washes, the dandruff packed my scalp and became itchy which is when the flakes would speckle my hair after I'd scratched it. I learned to relax it myself once my sister had got me going. I felt I was the best person to take care of my hair, so ritually, every two months, I got a relaxor kit from London and did my hair.

During lectures when I was trying to write notes, my hand shook visibly so that I wondered whether the person next to me and the lecturer could see. Outside of timetabled lectures, I attempted to do as many classes as possible hoping that at least one of them would offer some conviviality. Unfortunately not. In each extra curricular activity I participated in, it seemed everyone had been influenced by talk about me. I was ostracized or where a relationship with me was essential because of the nature of the activity (as in the Christian's union), people made digs at me by making an issue of what I wore, or implying that I smelled. On one occasion when sitting in the library head down attempting to do some work, I looked up to find that everyone had vacated the seats around me. Regarding my smelling, I could smell me too sometimes. A strong vaginal smell exacerbated by my nervousness in particular caused by the innuendoes directed at me during lectures. Glued to my seat to afraid to move a muscle for fear of attracting attention to myself sweat poured out of the sebaceous glands in and around my groin, which is what I decided was offending everyone. After a few weeks of this, I bought an expensive perfume, 'Amarige', and sprayed it on top of my clothes all around my hips in an attempt to stop the odour. It didn't stop the vaginal smell from coming through though. I broke up the term by staying with Richard at his house in Willesden, and spraying the perfume over my hips one night before going out, he started coughing and with a wry smile on his face he said that I'd put on too much. I decided not to go out after that. I had images of Richard and his friend doing things behind my back at the club, and this I didn't think I could bare.

At the beginning of the academic year, I got lifts to the poly from Mark on his motorbike. It was a wonderful sensation being on the back of the bike cutting through the wind, and Mark was friendly, not that I confided in him or anyone for that matter. I went jogging three times a week. I decided that getting lots of aerobic exercise was the best way of dealing with the stress that I was under. I overheard what I thought was a phone conversation between Dr Reid and Nadine about me. I mean *telepathically*, at least that's what I thought back then. Dr Reid was asking Nadine how I was doing and she was more or less telling him that I was fine. I thought to myself what a bitch. She didn't have a clue what they were doing to me here in Plymouth, or the stress that I was under. She had no right to say that I was fine. The impression I got from the conversation was that Dr Reid knew I could hear what was being said, but Nadine didn't and he was playing on this. Anyhow immediately after that conversation Nadine called me. I didn't tell her that I knew she had spoken with Dr Reid about me so we just chit chatted. A similar thing happened when I was in my room one day, the potent smell of my vagina infusing my nostrils and I overheard Fraser say in a conversation he was having with someone about me smelling, "A kind of sex smell is it?" I came to think of Dr Reid as my benefactor looking out for me when everyone else was against me. I decided he was the one that set up the relationship between Nadine and myself, him telling her that I needed help during my year out. This served only to raise him in my esteem.

In addition to Dr Reid's apparent benevolence towards me I felt the lecturers made a couple of attempts to contact me outside of lectures or at least to let me know that I was being carefully watched. On one occasion on my way home from Sainsbury's with my shopping, a red car pulled up further along the road, and I felt I was being watched by the person in it. I crossed over. It was only when I got home that I realised the driver was Dr Rob Ellis, a cognitive psychology lecturer and Rachel's tutor while she was at the poly. I didn't have my glasses on at the time so couldn't recognise him. I decided he was about to offer me a lift home and when I realised this, I could have kicked myself. I most definitely could have done with having some of the lecturers as friends, overtly. The second time something like that happened was when I was out one night with Mike and a few others. We were in a pub and Mike was with a blonde haired woman who he had worked with in his year out. Anyway toward the end of the night she was the first to leave, and then I left. Walking home I saw what I could have sworn was Fraser Reid with this blonde woman in a car, Fraser looking over at me. I felt he was saying that I was not to have the students as friends hence the blonde woman who was meant to break things up between us a bit. All of this conveyed to me it seemed at the time through simply a look.

My project supervisor was a German woman with long blonde hair called Dr Carla Willig. She was a new lecturer, gay (I heard) and beautiful. I gathered from George, the female students (not to mention the male students) loved her, saying she was trendy and good at her job. I found myself feeling envious particularly after I had attended a lunchtime seminar she gave in conjunction with a friend of hers, and noted the ease with which she spoke, nerves free. Given that I knew what the overall subject of my project was going to be about (i.e. interracial attraction), Carla and I had simply to decide on *how* we were going to study it. Eventually we decided on a questionnaire consisting of statements which subjects could strongly agree with or strongly disagree with, and three other intervening positions. So I devised the questionnaire consisting of statements like 'Blonde hair, blue eyes….what more could anyone ask for!', 'Black people are unfriendly,' and my subjects white and black male and female teenagers had to rate each statement on the scale ranging from strongly disagree through to strongly agree. I was really excited about my project. My overall aim was to find out whether black people found white people more attractive friends and partners than they did black people and vice versa.

I had a visit from Gabriela in my first term. She helped me find subjects to fill in my questionnaire, not in Plymouth I might add. I didn't think I would find enough black teenagers in Plymouth, so all of my subjects came from inner city areas in London. During Gabriela's visit we went to a night club and were invited to a party by a student we'd met at the club who had taken a shine to Gabriela. The whole time I was weary of the crowds both at the club and party because of people doing things behind my back. Gabriela on the other hand walked through like she didn't have a care in the world, and I suppose she didn't. She told me that Jessica was acting weird and that she didn't want anything to do with her anymore. She didn't go into detail. It was when I went home for Christmas that I actually saw Jessica for myself that I realized what she was saying. It was a day or two before Christmas day, I had spent the whole day doing some work and then in the evening Jessica turned up unannounced.

She looked a bit of a mess and smelled as we sat in the kitchen talking. Her clothes were ragged and she was wearing a wig that looked as though it had been in a fight. Not looking at me she said she didn't know what was going on. She went on saying people kept doing things behind her back. Just then my mum came into the kitchen, and as she walked past Jessica's back she made a gesture with her hands as if to say Jessica was mad. Jessica cried then touching the back of her head and said, "You see." I cried too partly for Jessica and partly for myself and told my mother I hated her and then told Jessica that my mother *had* done something behind her back. It was the uncertainty that did the damage I thought which is why I told Jessica what my mother had done. Whenever someone did something behind my back, although I knew they had done it, I couldn't be sure after all I didn't have eyes in the back of my head. I always wished my so called friends or *someone* would tell me so that I knew I wasn't going mad even if I didn't do anything about it. I figured it must have been the same for Jessica. She took her wig off. She had cut her hair short and thought it looked awful, hence the wig. I asked Jessica where she was staying, and she said she had a room in a hostel in the city. I asked her if it was clean because I commented if it wasn't we could go over there and clean up. I thought, apart from the carry on behind her back, there must be a reason she was in the state she was in. Unclean living spaces were certainly enough to make me feel uncomfortable and as though I didn't want to touch anything, perhaps it was the same for Jessica. Anyway she said it was ok and then asked me if she smelled. I told her she smelled of urine a bit (actually quite a lot), and she fell silent. I was heart broken at seeing the state she was in. I got some paper and jotted down a few things that I thought she needed to consider, among them being her feelings about God. At that time I thought when the world is against you can draw strength from God, which I suppose is what I had been doing. I told her that it was best if she took some time out and stopped going out, unless it was absolutely necessary. She agreed.

It seemed in the second term everything was winding up to some sort of climax. The malignance I experienced from others increased enormously and as a result my anxiety got worse. Subsequently I spent a lot of time trying to relax either running, practicing yoga or lying on the floor in my room. On one such occasion, I sat on the floor about to lie down and what I think was a tic jumped on my leg. Most certainly it was no ordinary flea. In a frenzy, I jumped up, brushed myself down and hoovered the room. Someone had been in my room, I just knew they had. I attended the few lectures that I was timetabled and with the rest of my time as was expected threw myself full time into working on my project.

At Easter I had intended to stay at Richard's place. I went out one day only to find I was being followed by someone in a white car. I told Richard about it who met me with the rebuff that I was acting strange. He also said in passing, "By the time they're finished with you Rose, I won't recognise you." I was too caught up in wondering why he wouldn't recognise me to ask him who *they* were. I was imagining an elaborate plot of me having to escape public recognition for some reason or other and therefore requiring plastic surgery. By the time I did get round to asking him what he meant, he simply said, "Nothing." On another occasion he commented, "If someone was doing something to me, I'd want them to kill me outright, not do to me what they're doing to you," without being specific about anything. I believe I was becoming a burden to him. Although he had this large beautifully furnished house, life for him wasn't plain sailing. He was having problems at work, I don't recall why, and he said he couldn't afford to keep the house as his cousin who he bought the house with had pulled out. We hadn't fallen out exactly, but he asked me to leave. Anyway I went and stayed at my sister Claudia's place. I didn't want to go to my mum's. For a start there were ants in the kitchen, and I didn't go all the way to Plymouth to do a degree just to end up back at my mother's place. It was ok being at Claudia's and anyway I had enough course work assignments in addition to my project to keep me busy. *My project*. My findings were what I expected, but not what I wanted. Black teenagers found white people more attractive than they did black people. Likewise white teenagers found white people more attractive than they did black people. My write up was relatively inaccurate as far as studies go, but seeing as Fraser Reid was now the head of department and oversaw the whole thing, he conveyed through Carla that it was ok. In my write up I pooled research from a variety of fields, and I gather I was suppose to choose one field and shape my study around that. To this day I am not sure, such was the nature of the supervision in my final year. Anyway the reason my study was unusual was because I wanted it to be as useful as it possibly could be to the black community and to this end it had to contain as much information as possible.

In the final term of my final year, for the first time ever, I actually cut my hair. Not terrifically short, but short enough. I can't say that it was my own decision either, I was kind of cajoled into doing it. First of all there was the behind my back carry on that got worse and worse which I linked to my dandruff, and then one Sunday at church, the bishop leading the service was talking about 'things' that were a hindrance during the sermon, saying if such 'things' got in the way you *cut* them off just like that emphasizing the 'cut'. Maybe he said it a bit more eloquently than I can describe. Now he didn't mention my name, but I suppose he didn't have to. There I was a social stigma who everyone seemed to know about through talking about me. Whenever anyone was making a seemingly neutral point, I immediately thought they were trying to say something to me indirectly. I thought to myself, it must be bad if even the bishop is talking about it. Then on my way home from church my mind spinning I considered cutting my hair justifying it by telling myself it would be easier to manage and that I could wash it more frequently and perhaps keep my dandruff under control. I discovered there was a black hairdresser in Plymouth from another black girl who I met around the poly, and I got this hairdresser to cut my hair in a straight bob the length of which was just past my ears. When I arrived she sat me in one room and went off to finish some business in an adjoining room. I thought Dr Reid was in there I could hear him so clearly commenting on what was to be my hair cut. He was saying to her not too short and intimating that if anything went wrong, there would be trouble for her. At first, I thought it looked awful, but after a while in the way that new hairstyles seem to, it kind of moulded itself around my face and I thought it looked pretty neat. I had an image of Dr Reid back in the psychology department amused saying, "she doesn't like her hair cut."

Cutting my hair didn't improve its texture as I deduced it would allowing me to wash it more frequently. In fact, nothing changed. My dandruff was as bad as ever and this only served to exacerbate my feelings whenever someone stood behind me, and wherever I went people made a point of standing directly behind me occasionally carrying on. So I thought I was psychic, and I thought the lecturers did to. I read somewhere that during episodes of extreme stress you can have psychic experiences and at that time, that's what I put my telepathy down to. I even saw Professor Jonathan Evans along with a few other lecturers carrying out a study on me on telepathy. In my minds eye, I saw them occupying a room in one of the houses opposite mine and although I couldn't see it clearly, I knew they had some sophisticated equipment. Anyway I fell asleep one afternoon in my room only to wake up having had the strangest dreams only I didn't think they were dreams at all. I heard first my mum saying my name gently and then my sister Claudia saying what were all her dislikes about me. I decided the lecturers had been in touch with my family because I was *special* that is telepathic. I called my mother immediately after and when I put it to her that she had been calling my name, she just laughed, but she didn't deny it. Now that the lecturers knew I was psychic I felt this was all headed to a positive end. Whenever they spoke to me there was a glint in their eyes and it was as if they were fighting off a smile. Shortly after I realized they could hear what I was doing in my room.

Yes, I decided they had bugged my room. I became so frustrated by this at one stage that I searched the room from top to bottom in an attempt to find the bug, not that I ever did. I couldn't even relax in my own space now, they were listening to my every move. To escape the tension, I went for long walks, and it wasn't long before I started being followed by white cars wherever I went. It was a while later before I realized that the police used white cars. Relationships around the house became more strained too. Often when I was in the kitchen cooking Mark and Darryl would come in to play cat and mouse with me. Caught in the middle of them, they would take it in turns to do things behind my back. Geoff found it all amusing. Darryl was taking some sort of body building drink and it was at about this time that I found I started building a lot of bulk in my body too. I hadn't changed my diet or routine so I didn't know why it was happening. I thought I looked awful, big and muscular, then I thought Darryl had probably slipped some of his body building drink into a yogurt drink I kept in the fridge.

The innuendos during lectures continued all designed I thought for me to analyse my background. During environmental psychology lectures Dr Tim Auburn harped on about the effects of overcrowding on your personality and amidst this lecture he mentioned something about having the worse garden in a street full of houses. Of course, I knew he was referring to me. Then in a theoretical psychology lecture, Dr Mike Hyland looking directly at me and nodding his head, spoke about the theory of rumours, confirming my thoughts that people were talking about me, and rumours had been spread. I pushed myself to speak up and contribute during lectures where previously I had remained silent too self conscious to say anything. I was still self conscious and nervous, but I felt as though I had to *prove* myself. Out walking one day by the sea front being followed, I contemplated suicide, jumping from a high point. I couldn't do it. It was Jules, a very posh girl from London who asked me during a break we had between lectures one day whether I had *any* money, meaning my family. Not only did I feel embarrassed, but helpless too. Her insinuation was that that is why this was happening to me, and maybe it was. To top it all, I got a letter from one of the girls I had met through Nadine inviting me to a church function in London. Working on a computer in the psychology department one day, the fire alarm went off and everybody had to vacate the building. It was on our way back in that Dr Reid talking to Dr Dave Stephenson said twice with his head turned toward me London, London, and from this I gathered that the letter was a cover for a secret meeting between Fraser Reid and myself. So I went along to the church function in London to find not only that the girls were hostile toward me, but there was no Fraser Reid. Fool that I was rather than deny that he had feelings for me, I thought maybe something went wrong, and he couldn't make it. Anyway at the church event Nadine wasn't present either. Both herself and her husband were now living in the north of London so had nothing to do with the east section of the church anymore. However I did meet a black female counsellor at the event who I believed had been sent by Dr Reid. She told me in the short conversation that we had together that I had passed my exams that I hadn't even sat yet.

The bathroom at Mark's house was arranged so that one end of the room the wall adjoining the neighbouring house was covered by a mirror, and at the other end there was a shower. Sitting on the loo having come on my period one day, I heard through the mirror end of the wall a man's voice say, "She's on her period," or something like that. The point was, they could *see* me. Following this I was flooded by male voices shouting me through the process of me going back to my room to put a sanitary towel on. My heart bled. Not in my wildest dreams could I imagine this happening to me. I couldn't get out of the house fast enough. When I realized they had probably been watching me since I moved into Mark's house, my mind flitted through what they had probably seen me do. I cringed when I realized they had probably seen me masturbate, and go to the toilet every day. In my minds eye they showed me an image of a man with ginger hair and somehow communicated that it was him that watched me in the bathroom. They were intimating that he was a coprophile.

Around exam time the stress I was under was ferocious. I barely did any revision, but I thought to myself, how was I suppose to revise in my current circumstances so nervous as a result of everything that was happening to me that I couldn't sit still long enough to read a book, much less revise. After a visit to the library one day during which I encountered the same carry on that is people vacating the seats around me, others carrying on behind me not to mention my thoughts that I was being talked about, I went straight to Dr Reid's office and demanded to know what was going on. He sat in front of me looking as though he'd just discovered a crown jewel, flushed with laughter escaping from him between words, "What are they doing?" he said emphatically. I drifted from his gaze then and thought about what the students were doing to me and couldn't for the life of me bring myself to tell him just in case he said I was going mad. Instead I repeated, "What is going on?" Thrilled by my presence and in the same vein he went on, "Well if you can't tell me what they are doing, I can't do anything about it?" As I had come to think that Dr Reid found me as attractive as I did him, I threatened him by saying, "I will leave," such I thought were his feelings for me. Anyway nothing materialised from that meeting. I went home to my room and cried and unbelievably in one of the houses opposite the one I lived in a group of women sat mimicking me crying, so audibly I think they could have been heard from the street outside.

As the exams drew closer the male voices increased in intensity usually restricting themselves to a commentary of sorts on what I was doing. On one occasion I bought some vest tops from the city centre because it was so hot, and when I had put one on, I was met by raucous cheers from the male voices. I thought that this was because they were pleased that I was revealing more of my body. One day as I sat thinking about all that I had been through one of the voices that I recognised was crying saying ,"You did it to her niece too." It was the addictive behaviours lecturer Dr Mark Griffiths. Fraser Reid responded, "You must sacrifice the few to save the majority." What I gathered from this was that the psychology department were behind all the foul experiences I had been through, and I was the unwitting subject in a social psychological study. Jessica too.

I refused to sit all of the exams. During the ones I did sit, the lecturers went out of their way to help me, making suggestions using props around me as to what I could write. At the end of the very last exam, I wrote a note to all of the students in the exam about the carry on behind my back and my dandruff. I said in the note, "if you want to look at my dandruff in particular, then make an appointment with me and I will allow you to view it unrestricted." Anyway just as I proceeded to read it out, everyone filed out chatting among themselves and ignoring me. The lecturers busied themselves with collecting the papers and looking at me said, "Is everything alright Rosie?" Extremely frustrated I cried, leaving the exam room with a few of the students who had also taken a year out. Back at home Mike Hyland's voice said, "It is all alright now." Funnily enough, even though nothing was said to me directly and nothing had been acknowledged, at that time, I *was* placated by this. It was Fraser Reid's voice that said I had better attend the year photo. If I had stopped to think about it one moment, I most definitely would not have gone along. Save a few acquaintances, I had been alienated by everyone. What did I want to be reminded of that for by participating in a group photo? I soon realized that the lecturers were communicating with Mark back at the house. Every so often he retreated to his room and it wasn't long before I could hear what they were saying to him sometimes. On one occasion Fraser Reid's voice, "Ok she knows now Mark, stop doing things behind her back," angry with Mark for tormenting me. I thought that Mark had a walky-talky in his room and that's how they were talking to him. With the exams over I thought my problems would be over too. I had concluded that the reason everyone was persecuting me was because they didn't want me to do the exams, or at least they didn't want me to do well in the exams, and if that were the case they most certainly achieved their aim.

Chapter 11: The Enemy Within

The journey home was what seemed like the worse nightmare I had ever encountered at that time. I packed just a few of my belongings and got out of Plymouth as fast as I could. On the train going back there was a young boy who reminded me of Fraser Reid. The voices told me that that was his son. The whole time I was in Plymouth, I never once considered whether he was married. All around me it seemed like everyone knew who I was and in the conversations people were having they were talking about issues that related to me, and all of this not mildly, but violently. I sat petrified in my seat trying my best not to allow my eyes or mind to wander the journey seemingly longer because of this. Inside, my mind raced and my heart beat so loudly and fast I could almost hear it. I wanted to fly off the handle, to scream, to tell everyone to leave me alone, but was too afraid to. On the tube going to Liverpool Street I sat in a carriage whose seats were almost all full. I sat adjacent to the glass panel beside the automatic doors. Two older women got on the train after me and although there were some spare seats, they stood on the other side of the glass panel next to me. As the train started moving they made faces at me so that I could see them in the corner of my eye. Every time I turned toward them, they stopped, averted my gaze and laughed at each other. I thought my head was going to explode especially when I turned to everyone else in the carriage and they sat wooden, one with a face painted like a marionette, and blankly looked directly ahead not moving a muscle. This ordeal lasted a couple of stops and then the older women got off of the train.

When I arrived at my sister's place I broke down crying telling her what had happened. Although she said she believed me she asked the question I anticipated from anyone I thought about telling what was happening to me, "how did you know they were doing things behind your back?" Telling her about everything was made easier by the fact that I thought the lecturers from the psychology department had been in touch with both her and my mum. I stayed at my sister's place, then on a visit to Barbara a friend of mine the day was going swimmingly until we hit Harlesden. We were driven their by a friend of Barbara's who was a lecturer she said at a sixth form college, then all the way back to the car, Barbara walking behind me gesticulated at me as if she were telling me to push off. I was so humiliated and this time by a so called friend. I cried when I got back to my sisters place. Perhaps not immediately after, but I did ask Barbara what that was all about. She denied all knowledge of her behaviour.

At my sister's place I slept in Ashley's room, the younger of her two sons. There weren't heavy curtains on the windows in the room so that at night you could see the street lights. Opposite my sister's flats was a tower block, and it was from this block that a huge amber light flashed on then off constantly directly into my room at night. I just knew it was intended for me. I felt as though I was going through world war III. It was Taylor my sister's husband who asked her to ask me to leave. Sometimes I heard them whispering in the kitchen, and I thought they were whispering about me. So I had only been there a few days when I was sent packing back to my mother's place.

My mum and dad didn't sleep with each other anymore, and hadn't done for as far back as I could remember. My dad occupied the main bedroom upstairs, my mum slept in the box room downstairs which was my old room, and I slept in the room adjacent to my father's which use to be my brother's room. The voices had taken to speaking to me directly often, usually when I was alone in my room. I thought they had wired the room, and had placed hidden cameras in the light bulb, too small for me to see, so usually when I was getting changed, I left the room and went into the bathroom, the living room or my father's bedroom. All the while, I thought the reason I could hear them was because I was telepathic and they moved the equipment they were using on me in Plymouth to one of the flats in Broke Walk where my parents lived. Jessica had taken a turn for the worse. She turned up in the early hours of one morning, the police not far behind her. She had been sectioned under the mental health act in hospital and had left the hospital. The police came to escort her back. Fraser Reid's voice was one of the voices I heard on a regular basis even though I had left Plymouth. His voice was soothing now having discarded the piercing tone he adopted whenever speaking to me in Plymouth, he was now the gentle giant, speaking as though some fantastic ordeal I had undergone had come to an end. Occasionally I telephoned the psychology department in Plymouth and spoke with him still insisting he tell me what was going on but never asking him to acknowledge that he were speaking to me on a daily basis almost. At such times he was callous urging me to see a doctor saying both the lecturers and my 'friends' were *concerned* about me. During another conversation he mentioned my name and address slowly and emphatically as though he were in disbelief that I was who I said I was.

I was awarded a third class degree, the only one in my year to get the lowest grade. To say the least, I was bitter. Only a week or two had passed when I got back from Plymouth and Sophie invited me to a lecture on 'Black family life and culture' by Dr Wade Nobles an African American who was also a clinical psychologist. During his talk I was met by the typical innuendos that I had become accustomed to. He gave an analogy using fish which I gathered was an offer of an explanation for what I had been through. He talked about salt water fish being more brightly coloured and beautiful than freshwater fish and that when a salt water fish was put in fresh water, the fresh water fish which were dull became jealous. At the end of the evening he said someone with a white car, reading out the car type and number plate, had left their car parked in a non parking zone outside. This was all the evidence I needed to tell me that he was colluding with the psychology department in Plymouth. After this lecture, whenever Fraser Reid spoke to me in my mind's eye, he was always accompanied by Dr Wade Nobles. Previously Sophie had given me the addresses to the Society for Black Lawyers and the Commission for Racial Equality. It was a few weeks after arriving back from Plymouth that voices I didn't recognise urged me to write to the Commission for Racial Equality. On the 6th July 1992 after a preliminary conversation with someone at the Society for Black Lawyers I wrote the following letter to them:

Dear Kehinde George,

I understand you have been allocated the advice officer in my case. The events I am abut to explain are lengthy, confusing and span a couple of years.

I am a psychology student at Polytechnic South West in Plymouth, and have just completed my final year examinations. My course has spanned a total of four years because I took a year out between my second and third year. The reason being that my emotional state was such at the end of my second year that I felt if I continued, I would never get through my examinations with the credit I deserved. By the end of my second year I was ostracized by practically everyone on the course, I was reprimanded for plagiarising a computing assignment, which I know was copied by over at least 50 % of the course. I was the only afro-Caribbean on the course. So, I took a year out for a break. At least I thought it was for a break.

In each job I had, both my employers and employees seemed to be responding to me in a consistent manner. It is only the events that have occurred in my final year that have made me realize this. Either they implied that I smelled (I bathe or shower daily), or that my hair was dirty (I'd have people standing behind me looking in my hair or just doing odd things behind my back), or that I was mad. I can only imagine now in retrospect that this victimisation was the result of poor references from the polytechnic. I know this is illegal. My employers in that year were:
1. *SAINSBURYS*
2. *THE TROLLEY STOP*
3. *SADLERS WELLS THEATRE*
4. *PAMELA'S WINE BAR*
5. *PYRAMID ARTS CENTRE*

*This happened so long ago, that I find it difficult to
remember the events clearly. All I know is that in each
circumstance I was victimised in one way or another and
the only possible link between these places of work is my
source of reference, which happens to be Polytechnic
South West, Plymouth.*

*But it has been my final year in Plymouth that has been the
real cause of my complaint. How I got through this year
and managed to complete all but one of my examinations, I
don't know. But I have.*

*At the beginning of each term, each student typically sees
his/her tutor just for a general chat about things, but
mainly to complete a form for administrative purposes. In
each of the sessions I had with my tutor Dave Rose, he
never once completed a form in my presence. I never
pushed the matter because up until recently, I did not
realize that this was the purpose of a tutor. A personal
tutor is assigned to each student to discuss anything
affecting the student's life. When I went to see my tutor at
the beginning of this academic year to relate my concerns
about the course, he was totally unsympathetic. Firstly, he
didn't give me the opportunity to say what I wanted to say,
and then he threatened me implying that I had better be
good because he was responsible for my references. I was
astounded, but didn't think to turn to anyone else. I simply
avoided my tutor for the rest of the academic year. Any
time I did see him, it was only for a few moments, and I
was never given the opportunity to express my
feelings/concerns about anything.*

*Everyone is allocated a project supervisor in their final
year. Mine was a woman called Carla Willig who proved
throughout the year to be inattentive and negligent. The
purpose of project supervisors is to guide your project
toward the production of a good scientific report. I spent
the first few months doing something that was completely
worthless to my project at her request. For the remainder
of the time I put most of the report together myself.*

*In practically every lecture I had, the lecturers
individuated me out in some way. They flirted with me by
either implying that I was cleverer, or more attractive than
the other students, or they suggested that I was mad,
schizophrenic or paranoid. By the end of the first term,
everyone else on the course hated me. I was totally
ostracized.*

*For the latter part of the year, the stigmatization increased.
I experienced mass hostility even from students I didn't
know. Sometimes I'd be working in the library, and after a
few minutes the students would have cleared the space
around me. Sometimes I would just walk into the media
services office in the library, and everyone would just stop
what they were doing and stare. Throughout the year, I've
had students doing things behind my back, things that
implied my hair was dirty or smelled. I've also been called
names meant to demean me in the street e.g. 'nigger'. The
hostility reached such an extent, that I stopped going into
the Student's Union.*

*I shared a house with three other male students, one of
whom is the landlord. During the whole year, they
mirrored events taking place around the polytechnic in the*

*home. My home has been a nightmare. We share a
kitchen, and sometimes I would have them doing things
behind my back, or implying that my hair was dirty, by
standing behind me and looking in my hair. They have
also implied that I smell, and on several occasions I
suspect that they have poisoned my drinks (I am a
vegetarian and eat mostly fresh foods). I've also been
sexually harassed by the landlord. On a couple of
occasions he has brushed up against me when there was
clearly enough room for manoeuvre. Shopping in
Sainsbury's had become a nightmarish event. I was
always on the receiving end of a lot of hostility from the
other shoppers. Spanning this whole period, I've had a
series of harassing 'phone calls.*

*People that I thought were friends of mine in London
suddenly began acting strangely toward me. I suspect that
they have been manipulated in some way. I also think I've
been followed during the whole of this year.*

*It is my belief that the psychology department have been
using me as a subject in a study (or series of studies),
without my consent. But that does not eliminate the fact
that I have been victimised throughout all of this. It's
possible that they have used me for a study on social
identification. This theory predicts that under
circumstances where the environment imposes category
differentiation (e.g. white people/black people) people
adhere to the stereotypes of their category. In addition
they have attempted to get black people to identify with
white people in circumstances where race is a prominent
category. If my speculations are correct, they have
succeeded (i.e. by associating being black with being*

dirty/smelly or unattractive in some way). All of this is speculation you understand, but it seems a valid explanation for the events that have taken place over this year, and in my year out. One of the guys I lived with in Plymouth was black, and his behaviour had been no different to that of the others.

Toward the end of this academic year, I approached the head of department Fraser Reid on 27 April 1992. I expressed my concerns about what was going on i.e. mass hostility, the lecturers responses to me etc. I was at my lowest ebb at this time. In spite of the fact he acknowledged all that I said, and admitted to knowing everything (whatever everything was),he said that there was nothing that he could do, and said that I had left it all far too late. He commented, if I had come to him earlier, that he may have been able to do something.

This weak admission from the head of the department that something more was going on played on my mind. I refused to sit the second examination and instead demanded to know what was happening. I spoke to a second lecturer Mike Hyland on 22 May 1992 whom noted all of my complaints. He admitted that there was a 'co-ordinated' response from lecturers toward me, but simply replied what was he expected to do. I left him feeling devastated. I did the rest of my examinations for fear of what might happen if I didn't, in spite of the fact that I was chronically stressed. I've been totally alone throughout this whole thing.

On two occasions lecturers that I have approached or that have approached me suggest I see a professional in mental

*health or my G.P. – the implication being here that I
imagined the whole thing. I don't want them to get away
with this.*

Etc. etc.

Of course I was careful not to mention anything about the
voices which I am sure would have seen to it that I were
not taken seriously. As it happened Kehinde George got
back to me in a few days and advised me to send my letter
on to the Commission for Racial Equality, which I did.
After sending the CRE a copy of my letter either I called
them or they called me (I don't remember which), and the
woman that I spoke to said we will have to arrange a
meeting. Only a few days later, she called me saying that
the CRE couldn't do anything for me as I didn't have
enough evidence. I was devastated. It was years later
before I learned that she hadn't followed procedure and I
was misadvised.

Bit by bit I was reminded of all of my past experiences, not
just those pertaining to Plymouth. The voices paid
particular interest to all of my sexual encounters especially
those I had with Perry. I wondered how they knew about
my past. Had people form my past been talking to them
unwittingly or had they been following me around for
some time? That's how naïve I was back then. The voices
told me how I was able to hear them and they me. All far
too technological for me to understand really, but basically
they can pick up my thought patterns ultra sonically they
said in the same way a sonographer can detect an image of
a baby in its mother's womb, only their equipment was
able to detect much more. It didn't just stop there either.

Practicing yoga at home one evening I got an itch on my arm and a spot appeared. The voices told me they did that too. It was some time before I realized that they could do this to anyone, not just me. They told me that they were doing this to me, because they wanted to get rid of illnesses like cancer and schizophrenia. The behavioural antics from others i.e. the carry on behind my back, they told me (years later) was a ploy that they had used against some of the Caribbean migrants in the 50's. Not to say that these realizations brought my torment to an end, because it seemed with each realisation the voices increased my stress levels. It was my sister Claudia one day who quizzed me about who the voices were. Their arms were far reaching it seemed, such that they could affect whether or not I worked, the media, and everyone I came into contact with. My sister asked me who ultimately controlled what we saw on the television and I deduced that the people at the very top were the Ministry of Defence. Having made recent enquiries I now know I was wrong back then. Anyway, it was eight years later that I narrowed the voices down to what I thought must have been the Intelligence Service. No other body could have so much control and be so secretive with it.

Eventually, thinking it was going to be another piece in the puzzle, I did as Fraser Reid suggested and went to see my doctor. I told them everything that I knew and when the doctor looked at me curiously, I knew he was going to say I was suffering from schizophrenia. I was referred to a psychiatrist, and put on medication that I didn't take. Still zealously health conscious I decided I was not going to pollute my body with drugs until that is I had been through years of being a revolving door patient, and finally realized that the medication was the only way to keep the voices at bay. I believe even my family conspired with the intelligence service as day by day while under my mother's roof, they behaved no differently to an outsider. In the early days, whether it was true or not I was bombarded with information and asked many questions by the voices. Once Fraser Reid's voice had gone, I heard voices from both the black and white community, male and female. They told me that each group was in a separate camp, otherwise it would come to blows. The black people were situated separately from the white people. Using my thoughts (they can communicate with you through thoughts), they told me that white people had evolved from a mix of dogs and the pre humanoid ape. Black people on the other hand, that is people of the African Diaspora, had evolved solely from the latter. I cried when they told me this. Why were they telling me I asked them, not that they answered. They went on telling me that the Asian community had also evolved from a mix horses and pigs and the pre humanoid ape. Indian Asians horses, and Chinese Asians pigs. Once they had told me, I justified it by referring to the tone of Asian peoples' flesh and hair saying it was pig like or horse like. I suppose the foundation for having white and Asian people as my enemies had been laid in Plymouth, and now they were building on it. They also asked me about the making of nuclear weapons, what caused lightning, the origins of language and the physics as well as the genetic transmission of colour. How was I Rosealine Mitchell to know about such things? However clumsily I tried to answer each question.

I guessed that they were asking me about nuclear power because the technology that they were using to control *everything* was nuclear. I don't know if this is absolutely correct. So there I was a black woman being courted by God, because that's who I decided they were eventually. They showed me that they could control every single thing about me from each hair on my head, to the colour of my skin to every personal thought, and it wasn't long before I realized they could and were doing it to everyone else to differing degrees. I begged them to change the hair of black women. I reasoned that the leaves of plants that grow in hot places are covered in a thick waxy cuticle, so it made sense that the hair of people that originate in these places should be the same. People of the African Diaspora should have long straight black hair, I told them. A white woman piped up, "that's dog hair". I didn't answer. I decided that the breaking and falling out of hair that was endemic to afro hair was what they called the 'fallout' of nuclear wars. I suppose the reason they were talking to me about evolution and colour too was because they had a big story about it, and this story wasn't to be found in our biology books or from the lips of any expert on evolution.

Like the famous line in the Shakespearian play of Hamlet that begins, "All the world's a stage……..," it seemed as though many people that I came into contact with were acting all for my benefit and sometimes to my detriment. It would seem also that this had been going on for some time, thus many people that I had formed relationships with were conspiring against me.

There was no let up on the torment I experienced from the intelligence service both internally and externally. Another

209

of the reasons they told me they were doing this to me was to put wrongs in the black community right. One of these wrongs they told me was that my brother was sexually abusing his daughter. I told his partner and she told him. He fractured my jaw the same day and I spent the next four weeks with my jaws wired together. They had lied specifically I believed to get this reaction from my brother as he wasn't averse to hitting women. My brother wasn't the only one who I experienced physical violence from over the next few years. When I had eventually been offered and settled down in my own council flat, I was attacked by Jessica. She simply turned up at my flat one day and with well placed punches assaulted me blocking every move I made. I was in a state of shock when she left. It didn't stop there either. Every time I went out, they got people to brush aggressively past me or tread on my feet without apologising, and it seemed it was all carefully arranged so that I couldn't retaliate. Either my aggressor was so fierce looking I kept my mouth shut for fear of becoming minced meat, or they walked on quickly so that by the time I was about to say something they had gone and the offence seemed too trivial to chase them for. Nevertheless, I wasn't agoraphobic exactly but going out had become something that I was beginning to dread always wondering what *they* were going to do next. It was all quite nasty. Whether I thought up this name myself or it was transpired through my thoughts by the intelligence service, I started calling them the 'Fat Fuckers' (abbreviated to FF's) and where I thought decisions had been made by women in particular, I called them the 'Big Heffer Brigade'.

Their antics both mental and physical were far reaching. As my room was next door to my father's one of the things they did was linked my father's coughing to my groin. That is, whenever he coughed the sound vibrated in my vagina so that I felt violated. Not surprisingly I began to resent my father. That wasn't the only cause of resentment toward my father. They had taken to punishing me with a severely brutal sharp shooting pain through my anus so that each time it happened I screamed out. I was convinced there was something wrong with me and was sent to Northwick Park and St Mark's hospital where I was examined. However, all was found to be in good working order. My father thought I was exaggerating the pain particularly at nights when he was trying to sleep. It went on for months before my doctors decided what they were going to do. Eventually they prescribed the anti-depressant Amitriptyline which is known to help with pain control. The FF's also interfered with my food. At one stage every single thing I ate had been tampered with in some way. For example I would by a bar of chocolate only to find on unwrapping it that there were finger prints on it or it looked as though it had been stamped on. They could anticipate which chocolate bar I was going to buy. In fact they could anticipate all of my actions. This culminated in what I thought was them getting people to interfere with my cooking. I felt as though some days whenever I cooked they would get someone to cook the same as what I was cooking in identical saucepans and then swap them over. I know it sounds bizarre and as though I had a screw loose but I was sure they did it because the cooking that they'd swapped over for mine was always slightly different, or at least I thought it was. But they can do that, get saucepans, clothes and even writing that is identical to your own so that you believe it *is* your own except for tiny noticeable differences that it has. It was all for a specific purpose I thought. They were trying to get me to loosen my inhibitions around sharing personal items with other people for some reason. Even if they didn't actually swap my food over with someone else's, the point is that I *thought* it had been and perhaps it was this that they worked on actually, making me *think* that I was sharing food with someone I couldn't see. Regardless of whether or not I was, it had the same effect.

These feelings escalated when I moved away from my mother's place in the spring of '94 the vulgarity of their antics taking on a new lease of life. Sometimes during mealtimes, they fumigated my nostrils with the smell of excrement or I was made to hear the distinct sound of a stool falling into a toilet bowl usually directly above my head. If I moved the sound followed me around the room. Speaking of toileting, when I tried to write in my diary or tell the FF's what I thought of them and they constipated my flow of words, a white woman made sounds like someone grunting, straining to pass a stool. This was followed later by black women doing the same. With my clothes, they altered their smell so that I believed I was wearing clothes belonging to someone else, identical to mine. Maybe this was all mental. Perhaps they altered the smell of my clothes in my nostrils or mind so that I thought they belonged to someone else. They even went as far as forging my handwriting and adding or distorting pieces of information in my diaries. *Or*, they made *me* write it unconsciously but the effect was the same, I believed my diaries had been tampered with. Unbelievable as it may seem, letters from Perry that I had previously burned, turned up without a scorch mark on them.

At one stage it was as if they had hired rent-a-mob, a bunch of the roughest and most aggressive sounding black guys. Whenever the mental torment of what was being done to me reached epidemic proportions they added to its malignance by saying, "Ya fucker!" or "Good job!" or "Biiiitch!" And then when I felt as though I really couldn't go on like this they shouted vehemently, "Now drop!" Whether these voices came from actual people or whether they were synthesized in some way, I'll never know I suppose, but I wondered how the FF's had reached the stage of becoming immune to another's suffering who was (I thought) physically so close to them. Soon, wherever I went I heard actual people say, 'Good! Or 'Good job!' in passing me by. I wondered what I had done to deserve such animosity. I soon learned that they didn't have to be close to me for their equipment to work. Wherever I was living I believed they set up a team of people in a nearby flat which is how they were able to dart in and out of my flat, me unconscious, and tamper with my belongings. They controlled my levels of consciousness as they could do to everyone and after a trip to St Lucia with my sister Francesca in '98 during which I experienced similar levels of harassment from others as well as mental torment, I realized that they didn't have to be close to me, to do what they did.

Amidst all of this, the carry on continued behind my back. This reached its limit when shopping in Mark's and Spencer on Mare Street one day two police officers standing behind me in a queue, peered into the back of my head. I thought to myself they've even got the police officers, our law enforcers at it too, who am I suppose to turn to? My hair was the source of much interest. Apart from the carry on behind my back, they got people to tamper with my hair while I was unconscious. They had started to make it break and fall out more than usual so I had taken to plastering it with grease. Occasionally I would comb my hair afterward only to find it was dry and brittle again, and stripped of the grease that I had put in it. In between me putting the grease in my hair and later combing it, someone had stripped it of the grease I put into it. The FF's also interfered with my sense of taste. Whenever I cooked a healthy meal it was tasteless, but if I ate junk food, they set my taste buds on fire. In addition not only was I subjected to the anal pain that had become typical of my daily life, but frequently I got abdominal pain too. My stomach would distend sometimes and I would get shooting pains through my abdomen. Some days I felt as though I had a clamp on my head which was fastened extremely tightly the tension about my head was so intense. I also became an insomniac very rarely getting a good night sleep.

As if I had nothing better to do, on a regular basis I believe they got someone to spread dust around the flat and this soon progressed onto insects. Not only were there ants in the kitchen at my mother's place, but in spite of my efforts to keep my room clean the FF's got someone to put beetles and spiders beneath the bin in my room and even on my bed. When I moved out, earwigs were scattered about my flat and often I found spiders on my dressing gown. Sometimes there was dog's dirt outside of my front door too. I was subjected to hellish noise pollution that I thought was caused by the family living above me. It sounded like one of the children was a gymnast who ran about the flat performing vaults each thump on the ceiling penetrating my body and my head. Whenever I went up to complain, a blonde haired woman called Jackie said it wasn't her or her family. It was as a result of this that I got into trouble with the police one day. I barely watched television because whenever I did I felt as though the TV presenters or news readers knew who I was and that I was watching and were often indirectly talking to me. On a few occasions I saw what I believed to be called holograms, live images of people or objects that aren't actually there. Once in Tesco, once in and outside my flat and once outside my bedroom at my mother's place. I wondered whether the life like images were a reflection on the retina of my eye, or whether they were images outside of my body which meant others were able to see them. I know it sounds impossible, but on each occasion, nobody else was present. In the same way they can enhance or denigrate your actual perception of someone by making their hips look wider or smaller or by making their hair look fuller than it actually is, the possibilities are endless. In addition when I spoke to people usually on the telephone the FF's interfered with the pitch of my voice as though they were children that had discovered a new toy. I burnt my thumb with hot water once and wanted to cry it was so painful. Instead they forced laughter out of me completely outside of my control. The whole experience was tinged with glamour as at various points I was made to feel famous African American actors were present.

I attempted suicide several times and in the beginning I was non-compliant with the medication as I was convinced

I was not sick and therefore didn't need it. I would save up the medication I was prescribed and then when I really didn't think I could take any more of what the FF's were doing, I would take an overdose. Obviously it never ever worked. I would end up in hospital sometimes because I called the ambulance myself afraid that I was going to be alive but delirious or in pain, and at other times I somehow simply miraculously awoke to find myself in a hospital bed. On these occasions on taking the overdose, I was determined *not* to be found. I locked the front door so that nobody could get in unless they had my keys and sometimes I put my bicycle in the hallway in front of the door to deter people too. When I awoke in hospital I asked the nurse how I came to be there. She said I called the ambulance and let them into my flat. I thought this was a lie. I believed someone nearby had the keys to my flat, and the minute I was unconscious came in with an ambulance and took me to hospital. There was never any sign of a forced entry. Once after an overdose, I awoke two days later to blurred vision, my body bent on one side as though a muscle was in spasm in my abdomen, my mind spinning and a heavy feeling in my body which made me feel as though I was going to collapse. *I* called the ambulance on this occasion. In spite of all the overdoses I took, I never once had my stomach pumped. I was usually made to simply sleep them off. I even contemplated jumping from the tower block that was adjacent to the flats where I lived. I would get the lift up to one of the uppermost floors and stand on the balcony tears streaming down my face begging the FF's to give me the courage to jump. They threatened me by telling me if I jumped, they would ensure that I landed safely, which made me cry all the more. They never did give me the courage.

I ended up on the psychiatric wing to Homerton hospital many times. I was detained under a section two or three times and on other occasions I agreed to be a voluntary admission to avoid being placed under a section. Most times when I was given the medication in hospital, I would slip it under my tongue pretending to have swallowed it, spitting it out as soon as I got the chance. When the nurses realized I was doing this, I was given a liquid form of the medicine or a depot injection. The medication was awful because it made you feel abnormal. If I was not twitching or able to sit still for long, then I was made to feel like a zombie my mind so slow that being gregarious was impossible and it made me sleep for most of the day. Sympathy from the psychiatrists usually depended on how young they were and the kind of people they had worked with in the past. In addition I often felt as though some were not who they said they were, and as a result of the conspiracy, were not actually psychiatrists. I was admitted by one such woman in the accident and emergency unit one day. She was almost unbelievable. When I told her that there were a bunch of people who were tormenting me to death, conspiring against me and were able to control all of my body processes she sincerely said, "Perhaps there are. Why have you come to hospital?" Her questions indicated to me that she had worked with women a great deal, and I was consoled by this. I told her I couldn't get the police to believe me and subsequently ended up on one of the wards. On the ward I caught a glimpse of what she wrote down about me in her report. She wrote that I was suffering from auditory hallucinations (hearing voices), was paranoid and the whole gamut of symptoms that go with schizophrenia. I couldn't believe it. On another occasion I was admitted by one of the women who were one of the voices in my head.

It wasn't long before I started going to church. It started with Sophie, who I had told all about the FF's and that they were in effect God. She was experiencing her own circumstantial and emotional turmoil and through this was drawn on cable television to the charismatic preaching of the Pentecostal church. She wound up going to a church on the doorstep of my flat, and each time she went she begged me to go along with her telling me that *God* (not my definition of God) could make it all better for me. So I went along with her eventually and although inside I couldn't shake what I knew to be true about the FF's, I tried my best to be carried away on the 'tongues speaking' tide of the followers of the church. Everyone in the church seemed vibrant and hopeful, perhaps I could be too. I never quite mastered speaking in tongues. Whenever I attempted it, it never did sound like the tongues that the other church members spoke in but I kept going to church hoping that *God* would free me from the FF's. At church I decided that the FF's were the devil and commanded them to leave in the way they taught at the church. They never did, so after a while I stopped going. A couple of years later when I was in hospital, my sister Francesca said she knew of church that held healing services. I went along asking to be healed of schizophrenia. Nothing happened. The church pastors encouraged me to make what they called a chain of prayers i.e. attending the church for several consecutive weeks at the same time. So I did and I also participated in what they preached, that is giving offerings and making sacrifices (usually giving more money) to ensure your miracle. In all of the time that I attended church, my beliefs about the FF's held fast although at times, my attempts to shake their hold of my life meant that they were not always at the fore of my mind. I thought the great thing about the Pentecostal church was the assurance that *God* could perform miracles in your life and turn negative events around for you. I had never come across this teaching in the Catholic Church; rather God was a distant entity who we hoped would alter the lives of those suffering for the better.

I believe my attempts to work were thwarted by the FF's. I filled in many application forms ensuring that I met the person specification requirements, and it wasn't until 1998 that I started being short listed for interviews. But shortly after arriving from Plymouth, the FF's told me that they were not going to allow me to work. I told them I couldn't care less and that I would educate myself instead. When the reality set in and I realized I wasn't being called for interviews, I tore to shreds my degree certificate thinking that it was worthless. In the intervening years I participated in many courses, not to say that it was easy. In each class I felt isolated socially usually because the FF's were interfering with my language skills in some way or I was generally set apart from the other students. I did a course in basic computing skills to increase my employability as well as doing heaps of voluntary work, and then did courses in woodwork, pottery, dance, guitar, massage and started a teacher training course in yoga but didn't finish because I felt so isolated and uncomfortable during the class. I also did a black studies class in Brixton, and in '96 finished one term of A levels in English literature, history and sociology the stress caused by the

FF's becoming too much to continue. During any spare time I had, I wrote songs.

My mother died on 15 March 1996. Before her death her health steadily deteriorated so much so that she needed a home carer organized by the social services to help with personal care. Near to her death she complained about pains in her chest and being breathless constantly. She died of multiple organ failure. My brother Curtis in particular was bitter about her circumstances before she died. He felt, as I wasn't doing anything, I should have been the one to care for my mother before her death. My father passed away six years later on 25 May 2002.

Chapter 12: Conclusion

I know what it looks like; you're thinking she *is* schizophrenic and as far as clinical observations go, from what I have said, that's probably true. But I would like you to step outside of what you think is true because you've read about it or heard about it in the media or learned about it from someone you know or the educational system and consider what I have said. Big Brother (or God) is not only watching us, but controlling our thoughts, feelings and bodily processes to varying extents, anticipating our actions and programming us to behave in certain ways the extent of which I can only guess at. I believe, as far back as secondary school, the FF's have involved various people in a conspiracy around me. I know my understanding of it all is perhaps a touch feeble, but I place my hand on my heart and say I am the layman in all of this. I do not have one shred of evidence for anything that I have said but I am convinced that all is not what it seems. What we believe to be *real* and *true* is not necessarily so. I told the FF's that with their power they could have created heaven but instead they had chosen to do the opposite. However when I thought about it I concluded that they probably have created heaven in pockets of the community around the world, most of us simply don't get to see or experience it.

Sitting in a ward in hospital one day I was brought the menu card by one of the nurses who pointed out to me that we were having rhubarb for desert. Suddenly I had an inspiration that these words had a secondary significance. Rhubarb is what actors say when they pretend to be talking in the background, while the main plot is going on in the foreground, and a desert is in addition to being a pudding, a hot place full of sand. Together I took this to mean that there was talk albeit clandestine about activities in the desert, and seeing as I had recently studied black studies, I took the desert to refer to the Egyptians, as that is where they had built the pyramids. I imagine this was no inspiration at all. I believe that information was transpired by the FF's. Now I haven't studied Greek or Latin which are often given as the derivative to words in the dictionary, yet following this I was then told by the FF's that sometimes groups of letters within words were short for other words, and sometimes acronyms. Language is extremely significant to our everyday lives and I believe the FF's have used it to create many iniquities. I am not just talking about class differences, but my experiences have shown me that where an individual is more eloquent than his or her colleague and has basic literacy skills in place, they are more likely to be higher up the social hierarchy than someone who is not and in addition they are likely to have a better sense of well being.

I learned in history, that whenever a country wanted to nationalize its people one of the things they did was to revive folk tales and myths which find their way into fairy tales. These tales and myths told stories of love, heroism and battles. I believe that these tales were often full of convolutions and inversions and the reason for this was to hide the truth, and this truth involved to a large extent black people. In English literature poetry and the literary novel is often full of irony and that's because poetic ballads and literary novels were part of the vehicles used like the folk tales to nationalise the community. Today the appeal of ballads and tales of love and heroism have been popularised through the media. White men and white women are almost always portrayed as the heroes and heroines and thus become national symbols for the white community. Subsequently it becomes ingrained in everyone's mind that 'things' aren't quite right unless a white man or woman is at the helm.

Meanwhile black people in the media very rarely get the attention that white people get. In addition where a black man is portrayed as a hero, he almost always has a romantic association with a white woman. While the image of white women explodes on the screens as the beautiful wife, the romantic partner, the loving mother, the aesthetic potential of black women remains relatively unexplored. I wrote in my diary after reading 'Ain't I a woman' by Bell Hooks:

15 Nov 1997

...........one of the negatives of the feminist movement is that it equates 'women' with white women by failing to acknowledge that the social status of black and white women is different and by referring to black women in the broad category of 'blacks'. White women are idealized by society and are fighting to be free from this. Black women on the other hand have never been idealized. Instead using the media as an example they are caste in roles that generally portray them as ugly wieldy characters usually at the fringes of the plot. This is mirrored by society where we occupy the tasks and jobs that no one else will do, kept

out of the private sector that offers higher paid jobs and are met by a glass ceiling............

In addition I am convinced that not only can a lack of eloquence be used to oppress individuals, but I am sure that so much of black women's oppression is tied up in our hair. I know that new relaxor treatments and well arranged weaves mean that this is becoming less so, but our hair is time consuming, difficult to keep clean and has a tendency to be dry and brittle.

It was Faith, the black girl who started up the African-Caribbean society in Plymouth who told me that some time in the near future the possibility of black people failing to exist as a race was a reality. Perhaps she had in mind the fact that there was a high rate of interracial marriage and romantic relationships in the black community, and if my final year project was anything to go by this trend is likely to continue if we find white people more attractive than we do ourselves. In addition, I believe that it is negative experiences with white people that cause black people to check their behaviour in relation to white people and become 'black conscious'. Bearing this in mind, should the white community become completely benign to black people across the board, perhaps Faith will be right. When the calluses on my feet itch, the voices tell me that this signifies the black community being desperate for romantic relations with the white community that is we are "call 'ouses" (or houses) the term house being used to signify the body.

No doubt about it, the FF's are behind all of our ailments and I believe that for the majority of drugs we are prescribed it is the FF's that exert their influence in our bodies. I think it is a great shame that these revelations about the antics of the FF's have to be coupled with insanity. I suppose it's their way of leaving the door open for any recriminations. I hope that this will signify the end to all our suffering as suggested by the song 'A design for Life', by the Manic Street Preachers, "… we are told that this is the end…"

I leave you with two ballads. One a poem by Keats and the second a song by Joni Mitchell. The poem has two layers of meaning which is common in the use of irony. On the surface, it is about love, but underneath it is about conquering foreign lands and sexually. The song Joni Mitchell describes as a love song that is a 'portrait of a disappointment'. Also, something to bear in mind that I learned in Black Studies was that in ancient African history they used women to represent the land.

La Belle Dame sans Merci.
A Ballad
(The beautiful woman without thanks)

O what can ail thee, knight-at-arms,
Alone and palely loitering?
The sedge has withered from the lake,
And no birds sing.

O what can ail thee knight-at-arms,
So haggard and so woe-begone?
The squirrel's granary is full,
And the harvest's done.

I see a lily on thy brow
With anguish moist and fever-dew,
And on thy cheeks a fading rose
Fast withereth too.

I met a lady in the meads,
Full beautiful – a faery's child,
Her hair was long, her foot was light,
And her eyes were wild.

I made a garland for her head,
And bracelets too, and fragrant zone;
She looked at me as she did love,
And made sweet moan.

I set her on my pacing steed,
And nothing else saw all day long,
For sidelong would she bend, and sing
A faery's song.

She found me roots of relish sweet,
And honey wild, and manna-dew,
And sure in language strange she said –
'I love thee true'.

She took me to her elfin grot,
And there she wept and sighed full sore,
And there I shut her wild wild eyes
With kisses four.

And there she lulled me asleep
And there I dreamed – Ah! woe betide! –
The latest dream I ever dreamt

On the cold hill side.

I saw pale kings and princes too,
Pale warriors, death-pale were they all;
They cried – 'La belle Dame sans Merci
Thee hath in thrall!'

I saw their starved lips in the gloam,
With horrid warning gaped wide,
And I awoke and found me here,
On the cold hill's side.

And this is why I sojourn here
Alone and palely loitering,
Though the sedge is withered from the lake,
And no birds sing.

Love or Money
(from the album Miles of aisles)

The firmament of Tinsel Town
Is strung with tungsten stars
Lot's of forty watt successes
He says where's my own shining hour
He's the well kept secret of the underground
He's indebted to the company store
Because his only channelled aspiration
Was getting back that girl he had before
He's got stacks and stacks of words that rhyme
Describing what it is to lose
He's got some just for laughs

He's got some for love
That mainline to his blues
Some to shed a little light on you and on me
Some to shed a little light on the human story

The wars of pride and property
The rebel Irish and the promised land Jew
Fighting behind his eyes and over seas
Wounded in action and no ceasefire in view
Brave reporters bring the battles home
But tonight inside that box
Just more bang bang ketchup colour to him
Just more Twentieth Century Fox
All because that ghostly girl comes haunting
Just out of reach-outside his bed
And she kicks the covers off his sleep
For the clumsy things he said
She commands his head-She tries his sanity
She demands his head-Tonight unknowingly

Vaguely she floats and lacelike
Blown in like a curtain on the night wind
She's nebulous and naked
He wonders where she's been
He grabs at the air because there's nothing there
Her evasiveness stings him
With long legs-long lonely legs
Bruised from banging into things
One day he was standing just outside her door
He was carrying an armload of bright balloons
She just laughed
She said she heard him knocking
And she teased him for the moon

"is one the moon, dear clown,
Tied to a string for me?"
He tried but he could not get it down
For truth or for mystery
He tried but he could not get it down
For love or money